Chronic Pain, BDSM and Crip Time

This book is a critical disability studies examination of the lived experience of chronic pain, engaging with and making a significant contribution to crip theory and the concept of 'crip time'.

Exploring experiences of pain and fatigue for people who live with chronic pain and based on narratives told through in-depth detailed interviews interwoven with theory at the cutting edge of critical disability studies, it demonstrates that our knowledge and understanding of chronic pain is incomplete without a critical disability studies approach. Through conceptualizing the concept of 'crip time' via participants' narratives of living with chronic pain, chronic fatigue, and variable disabilities, this book demonstrates how thinking about chronic pain and fatigue with 'crip time' exposes normative, ableist, assumptions underlying both how pain and the ideas of cure and recovery are understood.

It will be of interest to all academics and students working in the fields of disability studies, critical disability studies, crip theory, medical sociology, sexuality, and studies of embodiment, corporeality, and temporality more generally.

Emma Sheppard is a lecturer in Sociology at Coventry University. Her research interests encompass disability, sexuality, and time.

Interdisciplinary Disability Studies

Series editor: Mark Sherry, The University of Toledo, USA

Disability studies has made great strides in exploring power and the body. This series extends the interdisciplinary dialogue between disability studies and other fields by asking how disability studies can influence a particular field. It will show how a deep engagement with disability studies changes our understanding of the following fields: sociology, literary studies, gender studies, bioethics, social work, law, education, or history. This ground-breaking series identifies both the practical and theoretical implications of such an interdisciplinary dialogue and challenges people in disability studies as well as other disciplinary fields to critically reflect on their professional praxis in terms of theory, practice, and methods.

Accessibility Denied. Understanding Inaccessibility and Everyday Resistance to Inclusion for Persons with Disabilities
Hanna Egard, Kristofer Hansson and David Wästerfors

Understanding Disability Throughout History
Interdisciplinary Perspectives in Iceland from Settlement to 1936
Edited by Hanna Björg Sigurjónsdóttir and James G. Rice

Disability and Art History from Antiquity to the Twenty-First Century
Edited by Ann Millett-Gallant and Elizabeth Howie

Dis/ability in Media, Law and History: Intersectional, Embodied AND Socially Constructed?
Edited by Micky Lee, Frank Rudy Cooper and Pat Reeve

Disability and Labour in the Twentieth Century
Historical and Comparative Perspectives
Edited by Radu Harald Dinu & Staffan Bengtsson

Rethinking Disability and Human Rights
Participation, Equality and Citizenship
Inger Marie Lid, Edvard Steinfeld & Michael Rembis

For a full list of titles in this series, please visit: https://www.routledge.com/Interdisciplinary-Disability-Studies/book-series/ASHSER1401

Chronic Pain, BDSM and Crip Time

Emma Sheppard

Routledge
Taylor & Francis Group
LONDON AND NEW YORK

Contents

Acknowledgments

Firstly, and most importantly: Catherine, Charlie, David, Edward, Julie, Michelle, Natalie, and Rita. Without their generosity, none of this would have happened.

Secondly, my family and loved ones – my parents, Su and Nick, my brother Adam and sister Becky. My grandparents, Theresa and Arthur, to whom this book is dedicated – for confidence in the face of confusion. Gareth, who put up with so much. Alec, and Beth, for the past years. General Indigo, Holly Potato, Steeve, Melvin, Bob, Irwin, and Lady Thortoise – the best beasts.

In no particular order, friends and colleagues: Paul Reynolds and Allison Moore, for supervising and cheerleading. The DTTH collective, for holding my sanity when I wasn't using it. Sakura, Sarah, and Emma, for the laughter and immoral support. Sophie, Ellie, Annabel, Paul, Sayaka – for everything. South Norwood Knits, for friendship and dropped stitches. Kristopher Lovell, for every argument, and Elizabeth Benjamin, for every time I stopped by for 5 minutes and didn't leave for an hour. Kirsty Liddiard, Jen Slater, Dan Goodley, Ana Bê, Ria Cheyne, David Bolt, Emma Rees, Alicia Spencer-Hall, and many many others, for all the occasions to run my mouth. Colleagues past and present: Carrie-Ann Myers, Mike Saker, Rachel Cohen, Jonny Illan, Sarah Burton, Charlotte Butler, Cath Morgan, Ryan Scoats, Tom Murtagh, Marcus Maloney, Saba Hussain, Ashley Cole, Ben Dew, Tom Knowles. My students, who taught me so much.

Introduction

When I started this project – or rather, the research project that eventually became this book – I had some particular aims. I wanted to understand chronic pain, and ask what living with chronic pain meant in terms of receiving BDSM[1] or kink-related pain, and vice versa. Essentially, I wanted to shake chronic pain and see what fell out. The reason behind this seems pretty straightforward – and not at all academic, when I write it out. I live with chronic pain, and none of the critical theories or concepts or narratives of what pain *is*, socially and culturally and politically felt right to me. They did not feel right when I started the project, having been in pain for five years. Now, with closer to 13 years of pain, they still do not feel right, but Critical Disability Studies and Crip Theory have developed something that feels closer, more recognizable. Some of that has come from my own work, and a great deal more from the work of others.

A critically crip approach, which is the approach I have taken here, seeks to explore and destabilize the norms of ableness. For this project, crip gives space for narratives of chronic pain and BDSM together. At the root of this, I take pain – in all its forms – as something that is both *felt* and *discursively constructed*; two sides of the same coin. Discourse shapes feeling, and feeling shapes discourse. Exploring pain – exploring chronic pain and kink pain together – exposes how various discourses tell us how pain *should* be experienced, how those living without pain (and sometimes those living with pain) expect us to feel and behave.

Normative understandings of pain – informed by medical knowledge and medicine as discipline – do not adequately cover chronic pain, or pain in kink play. Disability and crip theories have begun to address pain, but do not consider kink pain. The understandings of pain in disability and kink are, at least at first look, very different, and located in experiences which are assumed to be not just different but *exclusive*. Disabled people are not expected to be kinky – and the initial response to learning that there are people who live with chronic pain who willingly engage with painful kinky play – even seek it out – is to ask why someone would want *more pain*.

Rather than merely queery the construction of pain as impairment and disability, I seek to expose how normative constructions of pain are a part of the performance of able heterosexuality. Thus, chronic pain and kink pain together,

DOI: 10.4324/9781003006237-1

not just asking why someone would want *more pain* but asking what these two lived experiences tell us about pain itself.

Facts and Figures

In terms of how many people live with chronic pain, Richardson's (2005) paper collected estimates of the prevalence of chronic widespread pain (which is defined as existing in more than one location in the body); those estimates range from 4.7% to 11.2% of the population of Australia. Conrad and Muñoz, in (2010), gave conservative estimates between 2% and 10% of adults in American, stating that other estimates went as high as 33%. Figures in the UK range from 11% to 16% (British Pain Society and Dr Foster Intelligence, 2011; Fayaz et al., 2016), with an estimate for the EU as whole giving a figure of 20% (Collett et al., 2010). Fayaz et al.'s (2016) meta-study of published articles gave higher figures, of 35% to 51.3% of the UK population, although the "prevalence of moderate to severely disabling chronic pain was lower and ranged from 10.4% to 14.3%" (ibid., 2016: 1); the participants involved in this research would fall into this latter grouping.

Incidence of chronic pain (or at least chronic pain reporting) is higher in women (Bendelow, 1993; Bury, 1991; Collett et al., 2010; Fayaz et al., 2016; Hoffman and Tarzian, 2001; Nielsen and Fernandez, 2010); in most studies of pain reporting since the 1970s, "women reported more severe levels of pain, more frequent pain, and pain of longer duration than men… women were also more likely than men to develop a chronic pain syndrome after experiencing trauma similar to that of men" (Hoffman and Tarzian, 2001: 13–14). However, when it comes to gender, this statement does not include intersex, non-binary, trans, or agender individuals – and I could not find statistical data estimating the incidence of chronic pain among non-cisgender/gender non-conforming populations.

Beyond gender, Fayez et al. (2016) reported that there is a trend toward incidence of chronic pain increasing with age; their figures for adults over 75 years of age were 62%, falling to 14.3% in young adults aged between 18 and 25. UK-based studies have reported a higher incidence of chronic pain in non-white populations (Nicholl et al., 2015); this is echoed in US-based studies (Hoffman et al., 2016; Trawalter et al., 2014). Other studies have reported a relationship between lower incomes or education levels and chronic pain – in that those with lower incomes and education levels are more likely to experience chronic pain (Nicholl et al., 2015). However, these studies did not differentiate between types of chronic pain, the severity of impact on the lives of those with pain, or the diagnosis they were given.

When it comes to intentional pain and sex, the numbers of people who engage in BDSM vary depending on what behaviors or activities are being defined as BDSM. Broad surveys of sexual behavior in the United States gave figures of 5% to 14% of adults engage in BDSM (Bauer, 2014; Janus and Janus, 1994; Reinisch, 1990), while Kolmes et al.'s figures go as high as 50% (2006). While all these figures are for the United States, it is not inconceivable that similar figures would be found in the UK – or that people living with chronic pain could also be engaging in BDSM play. However, there are no figures for the overlap.

Methodological Concerns

Cripping chronic and kink pain relies on narratives; here, those narratives were told through in-depth interviews with a relatively small group of participants. Small because I went for depth over breadth, and because I honestly was not sure I would find enough participants willing to take part – as the above figures show, it is fairly unclear how many kinky, chronically pained people there are. In addition, and just as significantly – honoring the stories told to me takes time. In the end, I had more data than I could cover in my thesis, and then in this book.

I have no idea if my participants are representative of the population. I know there are voices missing – the narratives of disabled people of color are missing[2] and whiteness, while a part of how the normative bodymind is constructed, is not a central focus of the project. The narratives of people with learning disabilities, and disabled people who communicate non-verbally are also missing. These limitations are wholly my own fault, and ones that may have required significant changes to the project beyond my capacities, and the resources available to me. In the end

I interviewed eight people, all living in England. Their experiences living with chronic pain are thus shaped by the specific conditions of the National Health Service, and, given when the research took place, the early years of the Liberal Democrat and Conservative coalition government's project of austerity, which has significantly impacted the lives of disabled people in the UK since 2011. The interviews took place in 2015 and 2016, over a period of nearly two years in total; the three interviews were spread over a period of about a year to 18 months for each participant. Three of the eight participants dropped out over the course of the two years, while the remaining five took part in three long interviews each, and kept diaries as well, between the first and second interviews.

The interviews took an appreciative enquiry approach; the participants agreed to take part having seen the initial questions which formed the starting points or the first interview. The flow of the interviews was led by participants – as was the format, with interviews taking place over email and video call as well as face-to-face, in cafes and pubs and over slow riverside walks. This flexibility aimed to take into account participants' varying capacities and energy levels – as well as my own.

Participants were found through my social networks, disability and fetish groups, and social media. From the outset, I was open about my own position as a person living with chronic pain myself. This undoubtedly impacted how participants related to me, and the balances of power in our relationships as researcher and researched. At the same time, in researching *both* disability and kink, being seen as either 'one of us' or at the very least a sympathetic ally is important (Priestly, 1997; Weinberg, 2006). The overlapping experiences and histories of disabled and kinky people in being objectified and pathologized – and the subsequent discomfort with researchers regarded as outsiders – meant that issues of power remained crucial within the interviews. I sought to balance power not just through adjusting how and where interviews took place according to participants' wishes and capacities, but also by explicitly welcoming their feedback on my analysis – where they thought I was wrong, their own views have stood. The research here has only occurred through their goodwill and willingness to tell their stories.

Participant Profiles

Natalie

Natalie is a white British cis woman in her early 30s, with Myalgic Encephalomyelitis (ME).[3] Her pronouns are she/her. She identifies as bisexual or pansexual, and is married to a man, who is also disabled. They act as each other's carers, with further help from friends and family. She has had ME since her teens, and did not finish secondary school. She is from, and lives now, in the south-east of England. Our first interview was carried out over email, the second by Skype, and the third by email. Natalie did not write diaries, but emailed me between the first and second interviews to discuss events and points she felt were important.

Catherine

Catherine is a cis gender but gender-questioning white woman in her early thirties, living in the South-East, where she also grew up. Her pronouns are she/her. She has a post-graduate level education and is currently working. She has multiple impairments (specifically: Ehlers-Danlos, fibromyalgia, and Asperger's syndrome). She is married to a non-gendered person, and her partner is the first person she has explored kink with.

Julie

Julie is a white cis woman in her mid-twenties, living in the south-east of England. Her pronouns are she/her. She is bisexual and has been into BDSM since her early twenties. She has POTS (Postural Orthostatic Tachycardia syndrome) and fibromyalgia, both of which developed in her late teens/early 20s. She has a regular play partner, and at the time of the first interview, several semi-regular play partners; she also plays with others at BDSM clubs. However, this changed to a single regular partner, with much less play in her life, as her impairments resulted in her being increasingly restricted to her house and her bed between the first and second interviews. She has a postgraduate-level education, and while she was in employment at the start of her interview series, she stopped working after the first. Julie's first interview was conducted over Skype, and her second and third over email; she kept diaries which she emailed to me.

Charlie

Charlie is a non-gendered, genderfluid, trans, male person, in their mid-40s, living in the south-east of England. Their pronouns are they/them. They are of mostly

European racial heritage, and have a mixed ethnicity. They identify as queer and as a switch, and are not currently in a conventional relationship, although they have lovers/play partners. They live with chronic pain, nerve damage, and a mobility impairment resulting from an injury over 20 years ago, as well as arthritis, Chronic Fatigue Syndrome and an associated Pain Syndrome, and autism. They are currently not in a position to work. They have been actively involved in BDSM since their 20s. Our first and second interviews were carried out face-to-face, and they kept diaries which we discussed, but that they preferred to keep private.

David

David is a white, heteroflexible cis man in his late thirties. His pronouns are he/him. He lives in the east of England, and he is not working due to his disability. He has chronic pain due to damaged cartilage in both knees, as well as the after-effects of a traffic accident several years previously; he is also autistic, and has dyspraxia. He has been engaged in kink since his early twenties, and is mainly a top, although he is exploring bottoming. He is active in his local scene. He is in a poly relationship with a woman. All three interviews were conducted by Skype, and David chose not to keep diaries.

Michelle

Michelle is in their late 20s, and is trans and genderfluid, polysexual, and a switch. Their pronouns are they/them. They are of dual heritage, and at the time of the first interview were living in the south-east of the UK. They are in a poly relationship, with one primary partner and two to three other partners. They have Asperger's, a chronic pain and fatigue condition diagnosed as fibromyalgia several years previously (although at the time of the interview, that diagnosis was in question). They also have chronic pain resulting from adjusting to surgery to correct being born with legs of different lengths. They have a university education, but do not currently work, although they do volunteer. They were raised in a religious household but no longer practice that religion. The first interview was face-to-face, and they decided to stop at that point due to ill health.

Edward

Edward is a white, cis man in his mid-forties. His pronouns are he/him. He has multiple sclerosis, and has used a wheelchair for the last 12 years. He identifies his pain as intermittent. At the time of the first interview, he was in an exclusive Mistress/slave relationship with a dominant woman, and identifies as straight (although he will play with men). He has a postgraduate-level education and is employed. He lives in the south-east of the UK. The first interview was conducted face-to-face, and he emailed diary entries to me. Edward stopped his participation after delaying the second interview, after the end of his relationship.

Rita

Rita is a white cis woman living in a small city in the midlands. Her pronouns are she/her. In her mid-30s, she is a university graduate who does not work. She identified as having multiple impairments that included diagnoses of ME, hypermobility, PTSD,[4] and ulcerative colitis. She lives with her long-term partner, who was present for the first interview. She identifies as bisexual and as a switch with submissive leanings; both she and her partner play with others. The first interview was conducted face-to-face, but after that she chose to stop her participation.

Key Definitions and Language Choices

The language choices I have made in this research reflect not just my standpoint as a critical disability studies researcher, they reflect my political – and personal – standpoint as a queer, disabled person. I use disability-first language ('disabled person' over 'person with disability') as my understanding of my experience and identity is shaped by the social model; disability is imposed upon bodyminds as a social process rather than an inherent, fixed, naturalized property of individuals.

In other aspects, however, I have broken with the social model of disability as a heuristic device. I do not split disability into 'disability' and 'impairment' – the process of disablement and the medical diagnosis – because I feel it is somewhat inappropriate given the difficulties the social model has with sensations and capacities such as pain and fatigue (Hughes and Paterson, 1997; Kafer, 2013; Rembis, 2010; Siebers, 2008). In addition, and especially given how chronic pain often comes with undocumented disability (Mollow, 2014) – disabilities not recognized or validated by current medicine – I recognize that impairment as a concept relies heavily on medical definitions and medicalized understandings.

The binary divide of '*body and mind*' is inappropriate in considering pain, and reinforces the separation of people with learning disabilities from disabled people as a whole; thus, I sought to find a term which works against both divisions. I have taken the word '*bodymind*' from Price (2015), who explained her use thus:

> because mental and physical processes not only affect each other but also give rise to each other—that is, because they tend to act as one, even though they are conventionally understood as two—it makes more sense to refer to them together, in a single term. I started using bodymind freely, mostly because I was tired of saying body-and-mind all the time, and unhappy about the implicit division created by the coordinating conjunction.
>
> (Price, 2015: 269)

I came across Price's paper partway through the research, and while the term has undoubtedly become significant in disability circles, it was very much a lightbulb moment. For myself, frustrated by the limitations of '*able-bodiedness*' (which can be easily read as excluding cognitive and learning disabilities), and the clunkiness of '*able-bodied and able-mindedness*,' which reinforces the binary of bodily and mental disabilities; I wanted a phrase that included without dividing. I switch between *abledness* and *ablebodymindedness*.

Within the research, I focus on chronic pain as an experience, rather than as a medical diagnostic category in itself; some disabled people experience chronic pain as a part of their disability, for a wide variety of reasons, while other disabled people experience chronic pain as their disability. I felt at the outset that limiting the research to a particular form or cause of chronic pain would place pain firmly in a medicalized setting, as well as limit the range of possible participants. I would perhaps define chronic pain, from my own experience, as pain that has lasted or recurred over a sufficient period of time that the person experiencing that pain feels it has moved beyond an immediate experience into a long-term one, which they may define as 'ongoing' or 'abnormal,' with little or no practical prospect of cessation.

Throughout the thesis I use the phrase *people 'living with chronic pain'* (or *'person who lives with chronic pain'*); this is a deliberate choice. As a person who lives with chronic pain myself, I feel that *'living with'* is a better descriptive choice than *'having'* or *'in'* chronic pain – in that while chronic pain has a massive impact on my own self-perception and my everyday lived experience, it is not the sum total of that experience; 'having' and 'in' leave less room for these nuances. It is also a deliberate rejection of the phrase *'chronic pain sufferer'* – a phrase I particularly loathe, which erases all other aspects of my life and implies that a chronic pain cannot be lived with.

I use *kink* and *BDSM* largely interchangeably; the former is, in my view, a broader term which encompasses a wider range of practices than those which come under the umbrella of *bondage and discipline, dominance and submission, sadism and masochism.*[5] It is also a more everyday term, and one my participants tended to use.

I have also used the first person *I* throughout. Trying to extract myself from the thesis, and maintain a place of aloof 'objectivity' would have betrayed my feminist and emancipatory research principles, and denied the interactive and deeply personal nature of doing this research, which I have detailed below, as well as in the conclusion. I reject the notion that objectivity is possible, let alone desirable. On top of that, I like the sound of my own voice.

Chapter Outlines

In Chapter 1, I look at how experiences of pain are underpinned by the discourses of normal; we have sociocultural norms of pain – which are shaped by medicine as a discipline and discourse – and in particular pain is positioned as ontologically negative, that it cannot be lived with and should not be sought out. We tend to conflate acute and chronic pain.

Chapter 2 addresses pain within Disability Studies; because of its medicalization – and conflation with acute pain – chronic pain is not particularly well included in the Social Model of Disability. However, a crip approach which explores normativities can be useful; in particular this approach eposes the lack of social recognition that there is for chronic pain, and the emphasis on cure, which is itself a part of neoliberal individualization and responsibility discourses. Responses to pain – especially stigma and abjection – are gendered and racialized as well as shaped by ableism.

Gender, race, and ableism play a part in Chapter 3, which explores disability and sex (which is not supposed to mix, according to the discourse); disability and kink is considered even less. Kink and disability both position the bodymind as uncivilized – in opposition to normative expectations of the civilized able body – but kink gives participants tools, including making pain and communicating pain, and space to enjoy sexual or erotic contact. I use Newmahr's four reframings of pain (transformed, sacrificial, investment, and autotelic) to understand participants' narratives, and critically crip pain in kink spaces.

Chapter 4 explores one of the theses which ran through participants' narratives: time. Time is important in how we define chronic pain (and disability), and so in exploring this I turn to crip time. Chronic pain is reliably unreliable, and participants needed (crip) time to readjust; kink play was a way to re-confirm the unreliability of their chronic pain. They also needed crip time to adjust to living with chronic pain itself. Pacing and adjusting to unreliable changes in capacities – and to decide when to engage in activities which impact pain and fatigue – also form part of crip time.

Chapter 5 is two sides of the same ideas: control and uncontrol. Control of activities and pain – through kink and pacing – was important, and for some participants, kink was a way into control, but also a way to feel a sense of engaging with their bodymind again, a positive re-establishing of selfhood. At the same time, kink was also a space to not be in control, to deliberately reject notions of control and civilization. For participants, pain is tightly controlled in kink play, but that same play also makes space to express pain, to be in pain without stigma.

Notes

1 This stands for bondage and discipline, dominance and submission, sadism and masochism – see Chapter 3 for a broader exploration of what this means.
2 One of the participants identified as mixed-race, but shied away from discussing the impact and intersections of her identity.
3 This is also known as Chronic Fatigue Syndrome, and thus the acronym becomes ME/CFS.
4 Post-Traumatic Stress Disorder.
5 The *D* and *S* do double duty here.

References

Bauer R (2014) *Queer BDSM Intimacies: Critical Consent and Pushing Boundaries*. Basingstoke: Palgrave Macmillan.

Bendelow G (1993) Pain Perceptions, Emotions and Gender. *Sociology of Health and Illness* 15(3): 273–294. DOI: 10.1111/1467-9566.ep10490526.

British Pain Society and Dr Foster Intelligence (2011) *National Pain Audit - Phase 1 Report: Organisation of NHS Chronic Pain Services*. November. British Pain Society.

Bury M (1991) The Sociology of Chronic Illness: A Review of Research and Prospects. *Sociology of Health and Illness* 13(4): 451–468.

Collett BJ, Betteridge N, Semmons I, et al. (2010) *Improving the Current and Future Management of Chronic Pain: A European Consensus*. Pain Proposal.

Conrad P and Muñoz VL (2010) The Medicalization of Chronic Pain. *Tidsskrift for Forskning: Sygdom og Samfund* 13: 13–25. DOI: 10.7146/tfss.v7i13.4147.

Fayaz A, Croft P, Langford RM, et al. (2016) Prevalence of Chronic Pain in the UK: A Systematic Review and Meta-Analysis of Population Studies. *BMJ Open* 6(e010364). DOI: 10.1136/bmjopen-2015–010364.

Hoffman DE and Tarzian AJ (2001) The Girl Who Cried Pain: A Bias Against Women in the Treatment of Pain. *Journal of Law, Medicine and Ethics* 29(1): 13–27. DOI: 10.1111/j.1748-720X.2001.tb00037.x.

Hoffman KM, Trawalter S, Axt JR, et al. (2016) Racial Bias in Pain Assessment and Treatment Recommendations, and False Beliefs about Biological Differences Between Blacks and Whites. *Proceedings of the National Academy of Sciences of the United States of America* 113(16): 4296–4301. DOI: 10.1073/pnas.1516047113.

Hughes B and Paterson K (1997) The Social Model of Disability and the Disappearing Body: Towards a Sociology of Impairment. *Disability & Society* 12(3): 325–340. DOI: 10.1080/09687599727209.

Janus SS and Janus CL (1994) *The Janus Report on Sexual Behaviour*. New York: Wiley.

Kafer A (2013) *Feminist, Queer, Crip*. Bloomington and Indianapolis: Indiana University Press.

Kolmes K, Stock W and Moser C (2006) Investigating Bias in Psychotherapy with BDSM Clients. In: Kleinplatz PJ and Moser C (eds) *Sadomasochism: Powerful Pleasures*. Binghampton, NY: Harrington Park Press, pp. 310–324.

Mollow A (2014) Criphystemologies: What Disability Theory Needs to Know about Hysteria. *Journal of Literary & Cultural Disability Studies* 8(2): 185–201. DOI: 10.3828/jlcds.2014.15.

Nicholl BI, Smith DJ, Cullen B, et al. (2015) Ethnic Differences in the Association Between Depression and Chronic Pain: Cross Sectional Results from UK Biobank. *BMC Family Practice* 16(128). DOI: 10.1186/s12875-015-0343–5.

Nielsen A and Fernandez J (2010) Journeys with Chronic Pain: Acquiring Stigma Along the Way. In: Fernandez, J (ed), *Making Sense of Pain: Critical and Interdisciplinary Perspectives*. Oxford: Inter-Disciplinary Press, pp. 45–54.

Price M (2015) The Bodymind Problem and the Possibilities of Pain. *Hypatia* 30(1): 268–284. DOI: 10.1111/hypa.12127.

Priestly M (1997) Who's Research?: A Personal Audit. In: Barnes C and Mercer G (eds) *Doing Disability Research*. Leeds: The Disability Press, pp. 88–107.

Reinisch JM (1990) *The Kinsey Institute New Report on Sex: What You Must Know to Be Sexually Literate*. New York: St Martin's Press.

Rembis MA (2010) Beyond the Binary: Rethinking the Social Model of Disabled Sexuality. *Sexuality and Disability* 28: 51–60.

Richardson JC (2005) Establishing the (Extra)Ordinary in Chronic Widespread Pain. *Health: An Interdisciplinary Journal of the Social Study of Health, Illness and Medicine* 9(1): 31–48.

Siebers T (2008) *Disability Theory*. Ann Arbour: University of Michigan Press.

Trawalter S, Hoffman KM and Waytz A (2014) Racial Bias in Perceptions of Others' Pain. *PLoS ONE* 11(3). DOI: 10.1371/journal.pone.0152334.

Weinberg TS (2006) Sadomasochism and the Social Sciences: A Review of the Sociological and Social Psychological Literature. *Journal of Homosexuality* 50(2–3): 17–40.

1 Pain

A Normal Amount of Pain[1]

Pain sits in an awkward place. Essentially, pain is considered a normal human experience, a marker for formative experience in normal development – but at the same time, the experience of pain is closely bounded by social norms and cultural expectations; pain is socially constructed. *Excessive* pain – whatever that is understood as, whenever pain becomes regarded as excessive – is considered dehabilitating and abnormal, and the experience of pain itself is regarded as dehumanizing and animal (Morris, 1991; see also: Scarry, 1985). In order to understand pain through a crip lens, it is thus necessary to explore the ways in which pain is regarded as normal or abnormal, to understand when pain crosses the line into excessive, abnormal, or disabling. This chapter will explore those normative understandings, think through these sociocultural underpinnings which shape how we experience our own pain, and how we understand and empathize with (or don't) the pain of other people.

Conceptions of what constitutes 'normal,' including the normal range of abilities, are relative from culture to culture and change over time. Perceptions of normal in much of the global North – particularly measurements of averages – are rooted in 19th-century science and eugenic attempts to describe and prescribe the ideal individual and society (Davies, 2006). Although notions of ideal or everyday bodies and lives existed before this point, particularly in philosophy and art, the development of science and, in particular, medicine gave rise to the concept of a normal body as a quantifiable entity, describable in terms of placement on a bell curve, from sub-normal to average, to super-normal (Davies, 2006). The quantifiable body, one that can be described as normal or abnormal, is not a fixed entity in time and across all societies; there is no rigid division between normal and abnormal that sticks everywhere and for everyone. What is regarded as abnormal and what is not is continually changing, as well as being heavily racialized, gendered, classed, and sexualized. In addition, as Wendell points out conceptions of normal abilities "depend on how much is necessary to perform the most common tasks of daily living in a particular physical and social environment" (Wendell, 1996: 16); what is normal, and what is ideal, changes depending on what roles those normal bodyminds need to do, and the resources 'normally' available to them. In the global North, we can take the idealized norm – the aspirant average – to

DOI: 10.4324/9781003006237-2

be in himself relatively rare: he is a white, middle-class, young (but neither a youth nor middle-aged), non-disabled cisgender man; he is heterosexual in preference and practice, vanilla and monogamous in his sexual habits, he is actively healthy not just in diet and exercise but at the genetic and quantifiable levels of weight, cholesterol, and so on; normatively attractive by the standards of his society, he is stably employed, housed, educated, holding the sort of political views that would be best described as reasonable.[2] He is unremarkably average and generic, but he is also extremely rare and precarious in his averageness – because to be truly *normal* he must be all of these things at once.

The measurements of bodyminds produced by the drive toward a population-level understanding of averageness served not only to provide a quantifiable value which could be deemed the statistical norm – such as intelligence, height, weight, and age of death – but also reinforced eugenicist ideas of who should and should not procreate, what Davies refers to as the need for "the state to attempt to norm the non-standard" (Davies, 2006: 6), and to create the perfectible human.

That eugenicist aim to 'improve' white Western people through 'selective breeding' required that certain measurable types of people be removed from the population, not just through the 'positive eugenics' of improved housing and sanitation, but through miscegenation laws, incarceration, and through compulsory and involuntary sterilization of those deemed unfit. This can be observed in such policies as that of incarcerating those deemed 'feebleminded' in the late 19th and early 20th centuries in America, which aimed both to protect certain 'idiots' from neglect (and their families from the burden of their care), and to protect society from so-called 'moral imbeciles' (Carlson, 2005). As Carlson points out: "as the definitions of feeblemindedness shifted to reflect the close association with a morality, giving birth to more than one child outside her marriage became a 'sign' of feeblemindedness … While the 'feebleminded" woman was a danger to society by virtue of her procreative powers, inside the walls of the institution she could nurture and protect her surrogate children," (ibid., 2005: 143) as she was forced to labor within the institution as a carer for other inmates.

I recount this in order to give context to this concept of *normal* which underpins everyday sociocultural, as well as medical, discourses of pain. For Tremain (2005) the description and prescription of norms is a key part in the apparatus of biopower; normality is positioned as desirable, but normal and normalized subjects are also governable ones; normalization produces a docile body, one that fulfills its role as a productive worker. For Best (2007), this is tied much more to a reflexive self, in that normality is something we apply to ourselves and measure ourselves against. In this reflexive application of normalization,

> normality … Is seen as a challenge, something that can be designed and produced, is a phenomenon that changes with time. Normality is no longer an external constraint that society imposes on its members; it is formed and shaped by acting subjects themselves. The conception of normality that currently prevails could in other words be termed *flexible-normalistic*.
>
> (Waldschmidt, 2005: 191–192)

Tremain, Best, and Waldschmidt all take their cue from Foucault, who when discussing medicine stated that it is concerned with

> a knowledge of *healthy man*, that is, a study of the *non-sick man*, and a definition of the *model man*... It assumes the normative posture, which authorizes it not only to distribute advice as to healthy life, but also to dictate the standards of physical and moral relations of the individuals and of the society in which he lives.
>
> (Foucault, 1973: 34 ital. rig)

These conceptions of what is normal (and thus what is abnormal) form a key part of discursive constructions of various forms of knowledge, particularly those around medicine, psychology, criminality, and sexuality. In the same way as bearing children outside of marriage once made one 'feebleminded,' being anything other than heterosexual made one either mad, criminal, or both; expressions of sexuality outside of the norm (as defined by the moralities of those with particular forms of knowledge) were treated in much the same way as disability itself (Davies, 2006; McRuer, 2006). While explicitly eugenicist aims may have fallen out of political favor, the impact continues in terms of the discursive construction of who is, or is not, disabled, and the continued inclusion of BDSM in the DSM.[3]

Norms of Pain

Norms of pain are, for this chapter, loosely organized around a few themes: context, religious belief, and medicine. Pain and suffering are often conflated in all of these discourses; suffering is often presented as incompatible not just with being normal, but with *being human*. It is impossible, according to these discourses, to develop or continue as a 'normal' or complete person, or a society as a whole, when you are suffering. There is, of course, room for exception, such as the productive emotional suffering of 'the artist' (Schwartz and Lutfiyya, 2012) or the temporary pain and suffering of pregnancy and birth – but overwhelmingly, suffering reduces people to animals, and counters the influence of (Western) 'civilization' (and indeed it is possible to identify moments when pregnancy/birthing is presented in terms of the animal, or the artist as uncivilized. However, discussing what makes pain and how we understand it problematizes a broad range of discourses and social constructs – including that pain is a negative experience, that is understood universally, and that it is rooted in either mind or body.

Few people can say they have never experienced pain – indeed, the inability to feel pain is a part of several relatively rare genetically-tied disabilities. A total inability to feel *any* physical pain from birth is rare enough that the reported figures for individuals with congenital analgesia are around the one in a million figure (Danziger and Willer, 2005). However, even individuals with congenital analgesia have reported experiencing headaches when under severe emotional stress (ibid., 2005); congenital analgesia does not affect an individual's ability to feel 'emotional' pain. In this way, the concept of bodymind becomes increasingly significant; the pain of emotions is experienced physically. However, in a normative context, we regard pain as *either* mental anguish or physical sensation; even when it is both, it is understood as having a root cause in one camp or the other; I want to delve into this in more depth later in this chapter.

The sensation of pain is, according to Seymour, "experienced as an attack on the phenomenological and embodied self" (1998: 8), resulting in a renegotiation of how the person in pain lives, in the spaces of their lives and in their self (Norridge, 2010; Scarry, 1985); pain cannot be experienced without the self requiring remaking, without a renegotiation of the phenomenological self. The argument put forward is that pain, no matter its cause, is negative and destructive (Siebers, 2006), the result of violence and damage that is experienced as jarring, as breaking the boundary of the self, the skin, and our perception of our lifeworld (Norridge, 2010; Scarry, 1985). This understanding of pain means that pain is always ontologically negative – it cannot be lived with or endured, and it should not be sought. Pain, and the breaking of the self that is assumed to come with pain, is seen as a negative process – whether or not the end result is a positive one – but an infinitely more negative one when pain is unsought and unprepared for.

Scarry (1985), writing about pain in torture, argues that pain resists language, and is thus not wholly understandable; we can only guess at whether another person is experiencing pain. Pain, in Scarry's view, is only undeniably real when we ourselves experience it – and we rely on the same language that pain resists in order to communicate pain; in English, we use metaphors and similes in the hope of finding common ground and shared experience. We talk of a 'stabbing pain,' a feeling 'as though we are on fire,' of being 'bruised and broken.' We need language to explain pain, and the language used is the key to unspoken – unspeakable – meanings (Bourke, 2014). Just as experiencing pain is a signifier of humanity – of being alive – being able to rationalize and describe pain is a signifier of being a *proper* human – in that the normal, proper human has the language skills and the knowledge of appropriate words to communicate a description of their experience, even if it can only be done once the urgency of acute pain has passed. The normal human can bring their experience within language through metaphor and simile, even if that language is clichéd and restricted. This expectation of, and ability to, put pain into language, to contextualize pain, to make it accessible to others, creates the normative structure whereby pain is further restricted to the animal and the abnormal; pain is ontologically negative. This understanding of humanity is at once normative and ableist.

Alongside and throughout the discourse of pain as ontologically negative – as incompatible with being human – we divide pain into two halves; there is chronic pain, and there is acute pain. This binary division relies on time as a diagnostic tool, alongside a medical understanding of pain (we shall return to medicine and pain later). In medical definitions, chronic pain is that which lasts for a period of more than a few months (Thomas and Johnson, 2000) and has ceased to be diagnostically useful (Morris, 1991), while acute pain is that which does not last, that is temporary, and is diagnostically useful. When pain begins, it is always acute, and only when it continues does it become chronic; in this way, all chronic pain is first experienced as acute – we assume that pain will soon fade away. Acute pain can be read as temporary – and while on occasion we may be in too much pain to fully comprehend that it *will* pass, those around us understand this pain as temporary,[4] as something which will end, no matter how painful.

Death is the ultimate end of pain, and death is often positioned as a form of *relief from pain*. However, when death stops acute pain, it is assumed to be violent and intimately related to the cause of that pain – while chronic pain does not *cause* death, it is not fatal in itself. Chronic pain is a side effect of disability, impairment, or illnesses which may or may not be terminal; the death of a person in chronic pain is regarded as a natural one, the end of a life that has been lived, while the death of a person in acute pain is a fundamentally unnatural one, an interruption of a life that has not been lived. Thus, time further divides chronic pain from acute.

Acute pain has, in addition to the expectation that it will cease through healing or death, a reason for being experienced; in medicine chronic pain is frequently posited as either without cause, or meaningless (Morris, 1991). There is a small but important difference between being *without cause* and being *meaningless* – to be meaningless, pain must not be instructive, it must not be warning of danger or damage, it must not be teaching us something, and chronic pain has long since ceased to do that; the religious discourses I will come to later position chronic pain as meaningful in particular ways. When chronic pain is medically diagnosed as without cause, it is because the original injury has long since healed, or there is no cause discernable to the medics at hand; the pain is experienced, but there is no injury, no underlying illness to respond to treatment (or an underlying illness that has no treatment, which is usually inexplicable, only vaguely understood, or of unknown cause, and all too frequently dismissed as 'psychosomatic')[5]. Sometimes, the pain resists medical treatment, or responds poorly. Chronic pain lacks the significance of acute pain – and thus its importance and urgency (at least for everyone except the person living with it). Despite the construction of chronic and acute pain being thus very different, it is assumed that the experience of pain is the same – that pain is an ontologically negative experience and an attack on the phenomenological self.

Contexts

The sociocultural context in which pain (and other sensations) take place affect how that sensation is experienced, varying from body to body, from time to time, and from place to place. Pain is not straightforward and – as discussed previously – requires explanations and interpretations that account for the sociocultural circumstances in which pain is experienced and expressed (Bendelow and Williams, 1995; Best, 2007; Morris, 1991; Williams and Bendelow, 1998). Communicating and contextualizing pain is important for pain to be understood by others, and even more importantly, to be recognized *as reasonable pain* when we express it to others. Pain is not the same if it occurs in different contexts – to work through some examples, if you stub your toe then the pain that results is expected, and while painful it is not of any great concern, unless you have recently had surgery on the toe. An ache in your legs is relatively unconcerning if you've been running for some time, but a stabbing pain when sitting in front of the TV is rather more concerning. A cisgender woman's period pain is considered largely normal, even when it causes her massive distress. The situations in which pain is regarded as normal – even expected – are highly gendered and racialized, with women's pain being regarded differently to men's, even as the pain of women of color is regarded differently to the pain of white women (Trawalter et al., 2014).

Bendelow and Williams (1995) recount that people have *pain beliefs* – individualized, personal beliefs that affect how pain is experienced and how we interpret our own and others' pains; these beliefs may or may not correlate with scientific understandings of pain, and are influenced by experience and personal history – essentially pain beliefs are sociocultural, and thus racialized, gendered, and abled. The three dimensions of pain beliefs which Bendelow and Williams summarize as "self-blame, perception of pain as mysterious, and beliefs about the duration of pain" (ibid., 1995: 153–154) affect everything from the immediate sensation of and reaction to pain, to how that pain is later recounted to others, and how upsetting that pain was. The experience of pain is inseparable from its emotional and cognitive significance (ibid.) – but despite this, the dualism of mental and physical pain persists. Research into culturally-constructed pain beliefs and reactions – starting with the studies of Zborowski (1952) in the 1950s[6] – demonstrate that bodies "cannot be understood as fixed or biologically given constants, somehow outside or beyond the constraints of power… [bodies] are themselves produced and regulated as distinct phenomena" (Grosz, 1995: 218).

While Grosz is talking of pleasure, the two are perhaps two sides of the same coin, both forms of sensation that are affected by culture and context, based on somatic sensation and emotion. If we accept that one somatic sensation is interpreted through discourse, then it is perhaps not so much a leap to view all somatic sensation as discursively interpreted, if not discursively constructed. However, those discourses affect how we interpret and process pain, how we express pain, and understand both our own experience and the expressions of pain from others. These discourses shape whether or not something is understood *as painful*, and then shape pain experiences and understandings – and whether pain in any particular context is normal or abnormal. Pain is constructed and construed through discourses that continually say that pain is bad; there is an implicit assumption in discourses around pain, that whether mental or physical or sought or inflicted, pain is bad and undesirable; we do not – should not – desire to feel pain, and seeking pain in and of itself, is abnormal and repellent. We engage all the time in these activities (and biological functions); we might even claim they are not painful.

Pain, Suffering, and Religious Belief

There is, of course, times when pain is regarded as a positive, or at least a necessary experience. Within medicine, and the various discourses of health, the exceptions are pain in childbirth, and pain resulting from exercise; both situate pain in terms of a temporary experience that must be gone through before the resulting reward. This discourse, particularly around pain in competitive exercise, situates pain as a sign of our own abilities or limitations – but particularly in terms of 'pushing through;' like the discourse of pain as needing context, this discourse is profoundly ableist, equating pain with weakness, and with not 'pushing yourself' regarded as 'giving up' – when those of us with chronic pain and fatigue may view 'pushing yourself' as a sign of both the ableist nature of the pace of modern life (Wendell, 1996) or as a need to stop and rest (Kafer, 2013; St. Pierre, 2015). This discourse, while overlapping with discourses of health and risk, overlaps significantly with discourses of pain and suffering in spirituality and religion.

Within spiritual and religious discourses, pain is often conflated with suffering; Schwartz and Lutfiyya's (2012) discourse analysis demonstrates that, for many religions, pain is a central premise of suffering. Across the major religious groups (Islam, Christianity, Judaism, Buddhism, and Hinduism), suffering, including experiencing physical or mental pain, is cast as part of life, albeit for varying reasons; this expectation that we all experience pain is a part of non-religious discourses too. Judaism and Christianity's discourses around the reasons for suffering are broadly similar – with the details varying between the various strands of belief or doctrine – with both religions viewing suffering as a punishment for sin, as a form of corrective education, and to deepen an individual's relationship with their god (Schwartz and Lutfiyya, 2012). Christianity, in addition, sees suffering and pain as purification, resulting from original sin – especially in the case of childbirth (ibid.). Suffering as a result of individual sin, in both Judaism and Christianity, originates in interpretation of the Hebrew bible. Within Islam, illness, disability, and suffering are viewed as the shameful result of deviance and sin (Hamdar, 2014), as well as – like in Judaism and Christianity – an opportunity for redemption and spiritual development.

Buddhism, in contrast, has one root explanation for suffering; it is the result of a selfish attachment to something, with relief to come from 'letting go' of worldly possessions and needs (Schwartz and Lutfiyya, 2012). Within Buddhism, suffering and pain is a part of life, with spiritual growth often equated with recovery from illness; in this way, suffering (and pain) is a spiritual issue as well as a medical one. "Buddhism suggests that suffering decreases and healing increases when we let go of wanting things to be different from how they are and instead move toward an acceptance of what is available in the present moment" (Schumm and Stoltzfus, 2007: 11). In a medical/psychological setting, this is echoed in the mindfulness therapy offered to people with chronic pain, as well as some mental health issues; mindfulness has its roots in Buddhism. This belief of the source of suffering parallels with the Judeo-Christian and Islamic discourse of suffering as a form of teaching the sufferer, or deepening their faith. In Christianity, with varying levels between the various branches, there is

> the pervasive… suspicion that sickness is somehow merited by sin and that a first step towards healing is the recognition of one's own guilt… In

> Christianity, as in Buddhism, healing is not marked by the absence of physical turmoil, but by the presence of resiliency and the quest to perform embodied acts of loving kindness.
>
> (ibid., 2007: 14)

The discourses in Christianity, Judaism, and Buddhism all parallel the cultural discourse in which pain and suffering is a source of growth (Bendelow and Williams, 1995), or, in terms of risk culture, the result of a particular behavior or inaction. Whether the discourses involved are based in religion or not – and in many cases I would argue that it doesn't matter, as a sociocultural discourse has influence regardless of whether or not it is explicitly religious, or acting outside a religious setting – ignorance of the actual experience of living with pain is the norm, with laypeople often unaware of what pain management might involve (Schwartz and Lutfiyya, 2012; Wendell, 1996). This, together with the aforementioned discourses, results in people with disabilities, impairments, and chronic illnesses

> [carrying] a spiritual burden resulting from a religious and social milieu that is suspicious of their spiritual condition. There is a persistent insinuation that chronic illness and disability somehow involve merited suffering (i.e. lesson to learn or result of sin).
>
> (Schumm and Stoltzfus, 2007: 10)

This insinuation that chronic illness is in some way merited can carry over into discourses of pain that are more strongly medicalized, or draw on medical knowledge.

Medicine and Pain

To examine the medicalization of pain alongside medicine as a form of knowledge, we can take a Foucauldian approach, positioning knowledge as a form of power, and the clinic and medical systems as forms of government and control. Tremain, when applying such an approach to disability, writes that "during the past two centuries, in particular, a vast apparatus, erected to secure the well-being of the general population, has caused the contemporary disabled subject to emerge into discourse and social existence" (2005: 5–6). This particular apparatus relies on a Cartesian dualism; the divide between reason and madness, sensation and rationality, self and other, and of course, sick and healthy, dead and alive (Turner, 1996) – and the aforementioned insistence on splitting pain into mental and physical.

Despite this dead/alive divide, it is the corpse that is at the center of medical knowledge, as Foucault points out in *Birth of The Clinic* (1973). As Leder (1990) observes, this contributes to the conception of the body as machinic, with fixable, replaceable parts,[7] where "the patient's own experience and subjective voice become inessential to the medical encounter" (Leder, 1990: 146–148). Wendell, drawing on this approach, writes that "the cognitive authority of medicine in the doctor-patient encounter gives far more weight to the doctor's metaphysical stance, undermining the epistemic confidence of patients in the importance of their bodily experience" (1996: 12). The positioning of the doctor as knowing, and the patient as unknowing, is supported by the process of becoming a subject of the medical gaze, where, far "from being a locus of self, patients' bodies are transformed into objects of scrutiny, organs in a sack of flesh" (Young, 1997: 11–12). This is echoed in Jain's exploration of cancer in the United States, which opens with an account of objectification at the hands of medical knowledge; "My flesh had become the pathology report – portioned, sliced, flattened onto slides, observed, categorized, and finally rendered into this emailable document" (2013: 3); in Jain's experience, the patient becomes an object that is incapable of knowledge, which only the medical gaze – properly trained and properly objective – can truly understand.

The contexts and meanings ascribed to pain within the medical gaze are relatively limited, and assumes that the reasons for experiencing pain – or describing an experience as painful – are equally limited. In medicine, seeking to understand pain is only useful insofar as a cause is sought, and pain is only useful for indicating that something else is wrong. Medicalization

> [encourages] individuals to interpret pain as 'meaningless.' In medical discourse, pain is understood as a symptom, indicated by the process at work, but in itself of no meaning. While acute pain… serves the process of protecting us, chronic pain serves no obvious purpose.
>
> (Best, 2007: 168)

Symptoms are a key part of medical understanding, as the physical manifestations of disease – but if we take Foucault's (1973) reading that little bit further, there tends to be the assumption that the symptoms themselves do not need treating, only the underlying disease – and therefore if the symptoms do not lead to a clearly identifiable disease with a straightforward treatment, those symptoms can go untreated. This reduction of pain to a symptom limits pain to the medical, and both Morris (1991) and Illich (1995) have posited that this medicalization of pain has led to a loss of significance and understanding – and thus made pain more of a problem; as Morris explains, "medicine unintentionally but implicitly depersonalizes pain by enfolding it within its machinery of high-tech prowess. It removes its quirky humanness and encourages us to forget that pain is not identical with illness" (1991: 174). Medicalization also places the control and treatment of pain solely within the medical sphere, devaluing and dismissing alternatives – or consigning them to the purely psychological. To understand how medicalization of pain does this, it is necessary to consider the medical theories of pain.

The basic, familiar, medical theory of pain, Specificity Theory, is the model of pain pathways found in schoolbooks; rooted in the writing of Descartes, with pain receptors, neurons, and the pain center in the brain receiving signals (Boddice, 2015, 2017; Morris, 1991; Williams and Bendelow, 1998). Specificity Theory primarily focuses on the sensory aspects of pain, where "'real' pain … means physical pain, anchored in visible tissue damage" (Williams and Bendelow, 1998: 157); this mind/body dualism dominated medical theories on pain (Morris, 1991), and although it has been added to in the second half of the 20th century, it continues to dominate mainstream medical knowledge. Bendelow and Williams (1995) outline these developments, starting with Gate Control Theory, first published in 1984, which stated that psychological and cognitive variables influence pain perception and response. Developed a couple of years later, Bates' Bio-Cultural Model built on earlier work on the cultural factors involved in pain thresholds, and added sociocultural factors to the original psychological and cognitive variables, and acknowledged that "social comparison and social learning within ethno-cultural situations" (Bendelow, 1993: 275) influenced how pain was perceived by individuals, alongside factors such as prior experiences of pain, anxiety, and the attention paid to the injury at the time. However, as Boddice points out,

> even though [theories of pain] began to change in the 1960s, we are essentially still living with [Descartes'] dualism in the way medicine is practiced ... Pick up a standard medical text book on pain and you will still find, as a sort of rhetorical Cartesian hangover, a tendency to label nerves that detect injury as pain detectors, which send pain signals to the brain. Such rhetorical slippages have been unsupported since 1965, but they persist and they continue to affect medical practice.
>
> (Boddice, 2015)

The Cartesian mind-body binary on which the medical conception of pain is built neglects the emotional aspect of pain. Subsequently, any pain thought to have a mental or emotional aspect is stigmatized in terms of how it is perceived and treated. Arguments abound as to whether or not chronic pain has a mental component – something that is frequently resisted by people with chronic pain-related illnesses, who see parceling chronic pain off to psychiatry and psychotherapy as a way of either dismissing their experiences as "all in the mind" (and therefore 'imaginary'), or as avoiding admitting that the medical community is not omniscient. In part this resistance results from their experience of having their pain stigmatized by medics. The development of theories that acknowledge the role of emotion and social factors, in the view of Conrad and Muñoz (2010), allows room for pain management strategies as second-string alternatives to outright elimination, which includes the integration of complementary and alternative medicine within a multidisciplinary approach to treatment and management. However, despite this apparent consideration for the role of the mind in managing pain, Gate Control Theory, like the wider biomedical approach, is focused on somatic pain alone – and does not give much room to pain that is dismissed under the label 'psychosomatic,' or give much in terms of assistance to those with chronic pain (Thomas and Johnson, 2000). As Bendelow and Williams wrote, the primary issue, once pain has been divided into 'physical' and 'mental,' is that:

> [whereas] physiological specialization for pain sensations can be identified, in that neurons in the nervous system are specialized to conduct patterns of

> nerve impulses that can be recorded and displayed, psychological specificity cannot be demonstrated in the same way. No neurons in the somatic projection system are indisputably linked to a single, specific psychological experience. Consequently there is no satisfactory definition which can encompass the diversity of perceptions [of pain].
>
> (Bendelow and Williams, 1995: 142)

More recent work, using MRI scans of brain activity, have shown that social and emotional pain has similar patterns of brain activity to physical pain (Eisenberger, 2012; Gunaratnam, 2014), leading to the potential for greater consideration to be given to the impact of non-physical violence – including social exclusion and marginalization – on bodies.

Pain is not, however, always viewed as negative even within the medical/institutional discourse;

> It could be seen as a sign of health, having a 'signal function' by providing a system of warning the body, and could even be perceived… as being productive, as in successful childbirth. [In Bendelow's study, positive] qualities of pain perception were associated with acute, short-lived, invariably physical aspects, although [there was also] the notion that character could be 'strengthened' by having to cope with emotional hurts. A central issue was that of control, linked to having knowledge and information, the lack of which gave rise to a sense of powerlessness. The more pain was associated with being chronic and terminal, the more negatively it was perceived and was inextricably linked with depression, poor self-esteem and mental illness.
>
> (Bendelow, 1993: 283–284)

Within this discourse, acute pain can be cast as positive in terms of its productivity; in other words, as long as the experience of pain itself remains negative and painful, it can be part of a wider positive event, or achieve a measure of usefulness that can construct the ability to perceive pain as positive.

More recently, a further medicalizing discourse has taken a foothold, where pain is a medical issue in and of itself – requiring holistic treatment, rather than straightforward suppression, while the underlying cause is cured (Conrad and Muñoz, 2010). Medicalization can present pain as a subject of medical-scientific research, resulting in greater support for patients with chronic pain – however, Conrad and Muñoz's (2010) optimism may be misplaced, or at least a little early in their assessment of the potential resources. As Wendell (1996) observes, somewhat wryly, doctors and medics don't like to admit when they don't know something – as a result of what she aptly describes as a hero complex – and therefore a person presenting with chronic pain (or other symptoms) that cannot be explained or cured are a problem, presenting as they do a challenge to the omniscience of the medical institution – which can result in dismissal of their pain, or active negativity or abandonment when doctors cannot 'fix' a person. Furthermore, the positioning of doctors as sole holders of knowledge about bodies rather obviously destabilizes the patient as being in a position of self-knowledge; when their doctor announces that there is "nothing wrong" or that their pain is "all in your head," people can cease to believe themselves, and begin to accept an incorrect judgment of psychosomatic illness, or dismissal without a proper diagnosis. For

> [many] people whose disabling physical conditions were not diagnosed for months or years [who] describe increasing worries about their own sanity and judgement … part of the relief of receiving a diagnosis, any diagnosis, is the confirmation by medical authority that they are not 'crazy' after all.
>
> (ibid., 1996: 125)

especially in situations where medicine, and the doctor, are figures of ultimate authority, and when medical discourses control how we can interpret our own bodily sensation.

Just as the heroic, knowledgeable, doctor is required to control their patient's body, they are also obliged to 'rescue' them from suffering – where suffering can be broadly defined as pain or illness (Illich, 1995). They must do so through diagnosing the cause of suffering, and then prescribe appropriate cure and rehabilitation, but first they must decide whether or not their patient's suffering is sufficient to merit rescue – whether they need, or are worthy of, treatment and rehabilitation – or if instead they must perform 'healthy' behavior first, through losing weight or making other 'lifestyle changes.' In this decision-making and diagnostic procedure, the epistemic experiences of the patient take a backseat to the knowledge of the doctor, who is able to assess the degree of suffering experienced by another with accuracy, thanks to their medical knowledge. Within this discourse, there is the "underlying notion that eliminating the person is acceptable, if that is the only way to eliminate suffering" (Schwartz and Lutfiyya, 2012: 29); the doctor's obligation is to end suffering, not to prolong life. The exception to this is the treatment of cancer, where prolonging life is the primary obligation (Jain, 2013). For the moment, I want to leave cure here, and pick it up again in the next chapter, where we'll take a crip lens to pain.

Painful Sex, Sexy Pain

In looking at BDSM,[8] pain, and disability, it is necessary to spend a little time on sex and pain (and sex and disability and pain), in order to interrogate discourses of what is considered unusual and abnormal, as in the case of disabled people's sexual relationships and activities, but also interrogating discourses of the normal – normative discourses of heterosexual romantic relationships and sexual activity. These discourses build expectations for non-disabled and disabled people alike; they are the measures against which non-disabled people hold themselves.

Within the heteronormative-romantic discourse that shapes the information and knowledge about sex, for cisgender women penetrative sex as a part of 'losing your virginity' is constructed as a painful experience (Jackson, 2005; Morris, 1991). This discourse "serves as a significant cultural resource in the negotiation of their relationships" (Jackson, 2005: 296) for young women, and the heteronormative-romantic discourse places young women as responsible for their own pleasure (and therefore lack of pain), but also for control over their male partner's libido and satisfaction (Jackson, 2005; Lindegaard and Henriksen, 2009). For women, there is a lingering discourse that heterosexual, penetrative sex will be initially painful or unpleasant, and that pleasurable sex is something which must be learnt, and that if they can endure the initial pain, they will then learn to like sex. Arguably this discourse is shifting somewhat, with an expectation that sex should be pleasurable for both, and both partners are responsible for pleasure within sex – but this sits alongside discourses which normalize and minimize pain during penetrative sex, positioning the penetrated person's discomfort/pain as of lesser importance than the penetrating person's pleasure. This normalization of uncomfortable or painful penetration can be a part of the expectation that heterosexual women will 'fake it' and simulate pleasure and orgasm – in ways much like performers in pornography – in order to support their partner's masculinity. Simulating desire and pleasure is frequently cast as both a necessary and regular part of heterosex, as a normal part of sex for women in the same way as discomfort is; this simulation is positioned as a part of a woman's 'duty' to ensure that the sexual desires of her partner are met, even if those desires (often phrased as 'needs') do not match up with her own. The emotional care work of faking sexual pleasure and orgasm can be experienced as pleasurable in itself – in much the same way as other forms of emotional care work can be – and is sometimes positioned as a part of maintaining a long-term relationship.

Although sexual violence was not the focus of the project (although the topic did come up in the interviews for Julie, Michelle, and Catherine in particular), it is important to touch on – however briefly – that sexual violence can include painful experiences; sexual violence is itself normalized by those discourses which normalize uncomfortable penetrative sex, especially those which present masculine sexuality as aggressive, conquering, and unstoppable. Approximately 23% of women between 16 and 74 years of age in England and Wales report experiencing some form of sexual assault during their adult lives, with 4.7% of men of the same age experiencing some form of sexual assault (Office for National Statistics, 2021; Rape Crisis England & Wales, 2022). Powell (2008) reports that 34% of young women in their teens and early 20s, living in the USA, report experiencing some form of sexual violence. As these figures are broadly similar to those from other Anglo-European countries in the global North it is therefore not unimaginable to extrapolate the following situation as being similar to that in the UK (Coy et al., 2013); 6% of young women report forced sex with their boyfriends, while 14% more report attempts (Powell, 2008). Taking these figures into account, it is therefore not difficult to see that while the discursive construction is of first sex as physically painful, pain associated with sex of many kinds (as well as rape and assault) can be a common experience for women on multiple different occasions over the life course.

This pain can derive from bodily injury and violence, and also from symbolic violence, which Bourdieu (1990, 2001) situates as a relationship of domination without clear violator or victim – in effect violence wherein the 'fault' is perhaps more complicated, violence was not explicitly used or threatened, and which pulls on discourses and relationships of power between individuals and social groups. Within heterosexual relationships symbolic violence can be exemplified by "young women who do not refuse unwanted sex because they feel that it would be inappropriate or believe that they are responsible for men's sexuality which once aroused cannot be stopped" (Powell, 2008: 173). While Powell's research is primarily focused on young people in heterosexual relationships (rather than 'adults' in established relationships), the discursive constructs, such as the sexual imperative, the gendering of libido and sexuality, and femininity, enacted by the young woman who does not refuse unwanted sex (Barker et al., 2015; Coy et al., 2013) are reinforced and internalized through repeated encounters, and become an expected part of heterosexual sexual activity. The experience – and indeed, expectation of – direct or indirect pressure to engage in unwanted sexual activity is much more common than physical force and verbal threats (Coy et al., 2013; Powell, 2008), and while individuals engaging in unwanted sex[9] may not experience physical pain in terms of a violent wounding, they may nonetheless experience pain as a result of the symbolic violence.

To turn to painful sex outside of sexual or symbolic violence, pain during or after sex is often positioned as a negative experience requiring expert, medical, attention. While penetrative sex is 'supposed to be' uncomfortable and/or painful at first, sex and pain are positioned as not 'normally' overlapping. For women, painful sex is often positioned in such a way as to be the female equivalent of erectile dysfunction and is more broadly positioned under the umbrella of sexual dysfunction, although there is no real consensus on what sexual dysfunction *is* in medical terms (Verschuren et al., 2010). Nonetheless 'normal' sexual function is tied to quality of life and psychological well-being, with the medicalization of treatment becoming increasingly the norm. When disability and chronic illness is included, the medicalization of disability leads to the assumption that painful sex must be a medical problem – rather than the result of a lack of knowledge or an issue of access. This is despite concerns raised around the lack of sex and relationship education given to young disabled people (Bahner, 2021; Barron, 1997; Liddiard, 2019; Rogers, 2009; Shakespeare et al., 1996). At the same time the asexualization and infantilization of disabled people leads to assumption that they will be not be having sex in the first place; while older discourses create a certain squeamishness about disabled people's sex in the medical field, those in the arenas of sexual health and sexual self-help (and to a lesser degree, sexology) can be equally as squeamish, and often ignore disability and non-normative sex (Bahner, 2021; Liddiard, 2019; Owens and de Than, 2014), and there is often feeling that disability is a step too far when talking about sex (it is also possible that researchers and writers themselves don't feel comfortable crossing into from one area to the other, due to a lack of existing discussion and writing). This squeamishness with sex can extend to those working with disabled people, and in the field of disability studies; discussions of sexuality and sexual activity are frequently confined to the twin spheres of 'sex education' and 'managing sexuality.'

Within medical knowledge (and as a part of the project of medicalizing pain), as Ruehleman et al. (2008) observe, there are a limited number of studies looking into sex and pain conditions; "those few[studies] have revealed: (a) that pain may precipitate sexual difficulties, and (b) that sexual activity may aggravate pain, sometimes leading to a reduction or complete cessation of sexual behavior, decreased satisfaction, or impaired performance" (ibid., 2008: 124). Figures ranging from 56% to 71% of pain clinic patients across four separate studies revealed pain having a negative impact on patients' sex lives (and by extension, the sex lives of their monogamous partners[10]); Ruehleman et al.'s (2008) own figures were significantly lower, but included people with chronic pain not seeking medical help at the time of the survey.

Significantly, Ruehleman et al state that

> greater interference with sexual activity is associated with higher levels of tangible support and impatience.... The person with pain who receives greater tangible support may be communicating messages of weakness and frailty to the social network, resulting in both greater support and a feeling of impatience in the supporter. These same messages may be barriers to sexual activity.
>
> (2008: 132–135)

However, while not disagreeing with these findings themselves, I would disagree with the interpretation, positing instead that greater need for support leads to a greater cementing of the perception of the person in pain as disabled; this means that discourses which infantilize and asexualize disabled people come to the fore, positioning the person in pain as no longer sexual.

Conclusions

A crip approach also reveals that chronic pain presents problems to these normative understandings of pain, which present very limited discourses about what pain is, why it occurs, and how it can be responded to. Those who live with chronic pain are often pushed into responding to their pain in ways which enforce individualism, deny interdependence, and leave little room to find meaning in pain, or make their own meaningful responses. Pain is regarded "as a systemic reaction that can be verified, measured, and regulated" (Illich, 1995: 137), with emphasis on its usefulness only for diagnosis, rather than a meaningful experience in itself. Illich (ibid) refers to cultures of pain in Western society as "analgesic" – as numb, where pain is regarded solely as something to be stopped, rather than considered as meaningful in itself. While I find Illich goes a little overboard in his rejection of medical systems and knowledge, there is something to be said for this conception of an analgesic culture. This is where Chapter 2 will take us.

Notes

1 Yes, I was watching *She-Hulk* when writing this.
2 See: Sedgman (2023) and Slater (2016).
3 Diagnostic and Statistical Manual of Mental Disorders, published and regularly updated by the American Psychiatric Association; homosexuality was specified as a mental disorder in the DSM until 1973 (and arguably not wholly removed until 1987). Having an interest in BDSM is arguably no longer classified as a disorder in itself, as long as the interested person feels wholly happy about their interest – this is the same shift homosexuality underwent in 1973.
4 Chapter 5 considers time in more depth.
5 See: Mollow (2014) and Wendell (1996, 2001).
6 Which while possibly insightful are also decidedly racist in tone; Zborowski divided his patients into racialized groups, and made gross generalizations – but he nonetheless demonstrated that reactions to pain, and pain beliefs were affected by wider social norms.
7 See also: Grosz (1994) and Morris (1991).
8 See the next chapter.
9 Unwanted sex is nonetheless different from forced or non-consensual sex and rape – in that unwanted sex is consented to, albeit unenthusiastically; while it is important to consider the role of consent in delineating sex from rape, it is also important to consider that consent can be given after persuasion and under duress, and is therefore not the sole indicator of that separation – and those who have engaged in unwanted sex may well not have experienced it as a violation of their bodily integrity so much as a chore, something that is neither pleasurable or engaging, but nonetheless must be done.
10 In all of these studies those experiencing pain were assumed to be heterosexual and in monogamous relationships; no mention was made of non-heterosexual individuals, those in polyamorous relationships, non-cisgendered individuals, or any combination thereof.

References

Bahner J (2021) *Sexual Citizenship and Disability: Understanding Sexual Support in Policy, Practice and Theory*. London: Routledge.

Barker MJ, Gill R and Harvey L (2015) *Mediated Intimacy: Sex Advice in Media Culture*. London: Polity Press.

Barron K (1997) The Bumpy Road to Womanhood. *Disability & Society* 12(2): 223–239.

Bendelow G (1993) Pain Perceptions, Emotions and Gender. *Sociology of Health and Illness* 15(3): 273–294. DOI: 10.1111/1467-9566.ep10490526.

Bendelow G and Williams SJ (1995) Transcending the Dualisms: Towards a Sociology of Pain. *Sociology of Health and Illness* 17(2): 139–165.

Best S (2007) The Social Construction of Pain: An Evaluation. *Disability & Society* 22(2): 161–171. DOI: 10.1080/09687590601141592.

Boddice R (2015) Pain: The Forgotten Emotion. Available at: http://beingmanly.blogspot.com.au/2015/11/pain-forgotten-emotion.html (accessed 29 November 2015).

Boddice R (2017) *Pain: A Very Short Introduction*. Oxford: Oxford University Press.

Bourdieu P (1990) *The Logic of Practice*. Cambridge: Polity Press.

Bourdieu P (2001) *Masculine Domination*. Cambridge: Polity Press.

Bourke J (2014) *The Story of Pain: From Prayer to Painkillers*. Oxford: Oxford University Press.

Carlson L (2005) Docile Bodies, Docile Minds: Foucauldian Reflections on Mental Retardation. In: Tremain S (ed) *Foucault and the Government of Disability*. Ann Arbor: University of Michigan Press, pp. 133–154.

Conrad P and Muñoz VL (2010) The Medicalization of Chronic Pain. *Tidsskrift for Forskning: Sygdom og Samfund* 13: 13–25. DOI: 10.7146/tfss.v7i13.4147.

Coy M, Kelly L, Elvines F, et al. (2013) *"Sex Without Consent, I Suppose That Is Rape": How Young People in England Understand Sexual Consent: A Report Commissioned for the Office of the Children's Commissioner's Inquiry into Child Sexual Exploitation in Gangs and Groups*. Office of the Children's Commissioner.

Danziger N and Willer J-C (2005) Tension-Type Headache as the Unique Pain Experience of a Patient with Congenital Insensitivity to Pain. *Pain* 117: 478–483. DOI: 10.1016/j.pain.2005.07.012.

Davies LJ (2006) Constructing Normalcy: The Bell Curve, the Norm, and the Invention of the Disabled Body in the Nineteenth Century. In: Davies LJ (ed) *The Disability Studies Reader*. 2nd ed. Abingdon: Routledge, pp. 3–16.

Eisenberger NI (2012) Broken Hearts and Broken Bones: A Neural Perspective on the Similarities Between Social and Physical Pain. *Current Directions in Psychological Science* 21(1): 42–47. DOI: 10.1177/0963721411429455.

Foucault M (1973) *The Birth of the Clinic: An Archaeology of Medical Perception* (trans. AM Sheridan). London: Tavistock Publications Ltd.

Grosz EA (1994) *Volatile Bodies: Towards a Corporeal Feminism*. Bloomington: Indiana University Press.

Grosz EA (1995) *Space, Time, and Perversion: Essays on the Politics of Bodies*. London: Routledge.

Gunaratnam Y (2014) Morbid Mixtures: Hybridity, Pain and Transnational Dying. *Subjectivity* 7: 74–91. DOI: 10.1057/sub.2013.21.

Hamdar A (2014) *The Female Suffering Body: Illness and Disability in Modern Arabic Literature*. Syracuse, NY: Syracuse University Press.

Illich I (1995) *Limits to Medicine: Medical Nemesis, the Expropriation of Health*. London: Marion Boyars Publishers Ltd.

Jackson S (2005) 'Dear Girlfriend…': Constructions of Sexual Health Problems and Sexual Identities in Letters to a Teenage Magazine. *Sexualities* 8(3): 282–305.

Jain SL (2013) *Malignant: How Cancer Becomes Us*. Oakland: University of California Press.

Kafer A (2013) *Feminist, Queer, Crip*. Bloomington and Indianapolis: Indiana University Press.

Leder D (1990) *The Absent Body*. Chicago, IL: University of Chicago Press.

Liddiard K (2019) *The Intimate Lives of Disabled People*. Abingdon: Routledge.

Lindegaard MR and Henriksen A-K (2009) Chapter 2: Sexually Active Virgins: Negotiating Adolescent Femininity: Colour and Safety in Cape Town. In: Donnan H and Magowan F (eds) *Transgressive Sex: Subversion and Control in Erotic Encounters*. e-book. Fertility, Reproduction and Society. New York: Berghahn Books.

McRuer R (2006) *Crip Theory: Cultural Signs of Queerness and Disability*. New York: NYU Press.

Mollow A (2014) Criphystemologies: What Disability Theory Needs to Know about Hysteria. *Journal of Literary & Cultural Disability Studies* 8(2): 185–201. DOI: 10.3828/jlcds.2014.15.

Morris DB (1991) *The Culture of Pain*. Berkeley: University of California Press.

Norridge Z (2010) Perceptions of Pain in Contemporary Zimbabwean Literature: Personal and Public Narratives in Yvonne Vera's The Stone Virgins. In: Lange I and Norridge Z (eds) *Illness, Bodies and Contexts: Interdisciplinary Perspectives*. Oxford: Inter-disciplinary Press, pp. 27–36.

Office for National Statistics (2021) Sexual Offences Prevalence and Trends, England and Wales: Year Ending March 2020. Available at: https://www.ons.gov.uk/peoplepopulationandcommunity/crimeandjustice/articles/sexualoffencesprevalenceandtrendsenglandandwales/latest (accessed 29 December 2022).

Owens T and de Than C (2014) *Supporting Disabled People with Their Sexual Lives: A Clear Guide for Health and Social Care Professionals*. London: Jessica Kingsley Publishers.

Powell A (2008) Amor Fati?: Gender Habitus and Young People's Negotiation of (Hetero) Sexual Consent. *Journal of Sociology* 44(2): 167–184.

Rape Crisis England & Wales (2022) Statistics about Sexual Violence and Abuse. Available at: https://rapecrisis.org.uk/get-informed/statistics-sexual-violence/ (accessed 29 December 2022).

Rogers C (2009) (S)excerpts from a Life Told: Sex, Gender and Learning Disability. *Sexualities* 12(3): 270–288.

Ruehlman LS, Karoly P and Taylor A (2008) Perceptions of Chronic Pain's Interference with Sexual Functioning: the Role of Gender, Treatment Status, and Psychosocial Factors. *Sexuality and Disability* 26: 123–136.

Scarry E (1985) *The Body in Pain: The Making and Unmaking of the World*. New York: Oxford University Press.

Schumm DY and Stoltzfus M (2007) Chronic Illness and Disability. *Journal of Religion, Disability and Health* 11(3): 5–21.

Schwartz KD and Lutfiyya ZM (2012) 'In Pain Waiting to Die': Everyday Understandings of Suffering. *Palliative and Supportive Care* 10: 27–36. DOI: 10.1017/S1478951511000551.

Sedgman K (2023) *On Being Unreasonable*. S.l.: Faber and Faber.

Seymour W (1998) *Remaking the Body: Rehabilitation and Change*. St Leonards: Unwin.

Shakespeare T, Gillespie-Sells K and Davies D (1996) *The Sexual Politics of Disability: Untold Desires*. London and New York: Cassell.

Siebers T (2006) Disability in Theory: From Social Constructionism to the New Realism of the Body. In: Davies LJ (ed) *The Disability Studies Reader*. 2nd ed. Abingdon: Routledge, pp. 173–183.

Slater J (2016) *Youth and Disability: A Challenge to Mr Reasonable*. London: Routledge.

St. Pierre J (2015) Distending Straight-Masculine Time: A Phenomenology of the Disabled Speaking Body. *Hypatia* 30(1): 49–65. DOI: 10.1111/hypa.12128.

Thomas SP and Johnson M (2000) A Phenomenologic Study of Chronic Pain. *Western Journal of Nursing Research* 22(6): 683–705.

Trawalter S, Hoffman KM and Waytz A (2014) Racial Bias in Perceptions of Others' Pain. *PLoS ONE* 11(3). DOI: 10.1371/journal.pone.0152334.

Tremain S (2005) Foucault, Governmentality, and Critical Disability Theory. In: Tremain S (ed) *Foucault and the Government of Disability*. Ann Arbor: University of Michigan Press, pp. 1–24.

Turner BS (1996) *The Body and Society*. 2nd ed. London: Sage.

Verschuren JEA, Enzlin P, Dijkstra PU, et al. (2010) Chronic Disease and Sexuality: A Generic Conceptual Framework. *Journal of Sex Research* 47(2–3): 153–170.

Waldschmidt A (2005) Who Is Normal? Who Is Deviant? 'Normality' and 'Risk' in Genetic Diagnostics and Counselling. In: Tremain S (ed) *Foucault and the Government of Disability*. Ann Arbor: University of Michigan Press, pp. 191–207.

Wendell S (1996) *The Rejected Body: Feminist Philosophical Reflections on Disability*. New York: Routledge.

Wendell S (2001) Unhealthy Disabled: Treating Chronic Illness as Disabilities. *Hypatia* 16(4): 17–33.

Williams SJ and Bendelow G (1998) *The Lived Body: Sociological Themes, Embodied Issues.* Abingdon: Routledge.

Young K (1997) *Presence in the Flesh: The Body in Medicine.* Cambridge, MA: Harvard University Press.

Zborowski M (1952) Cultural Components in Responses to Pain. *Journal of Social Issues* 8(4): 16–30.

2 Cripping Pain

Introduction

In this chapter I will start to quote from participants.[1] Bringing in their own voices, rather than merely my interpretations – regardless of my position as a person living with chronic pain – recognizes the importance here of self-representation, and of placing the role of expert firmly in *their* hands. They are the expert knowers – the ones best placed to explain their own experiences. When I misinterpreted or misunderstood, their explanation has stood – and they have told me if they agree with what I am writing.

Pain and Disability

Without wishing to rehash an explanation of the social model before digging into a crip reading of pain, it becomes important to explore how pain is understood within the frames of various models of disability. Within the social model impairment is understood through a medical frame arguably in much the same way the medical model understands disability, and experience of embodied impairment is either ignored or rather awkwardly dealt with – particularly once we dig into a more conceptual understanding of embodied experience (see Hughes and Paterson, 1997). Pain in particular is considered a largely medical or psychological problem within the social model, due to the perception that pain is either sensory and therefore needs to be treated medically (Seymour, 1998), or is psychological and therefore needs to be treated by psychologists (Wendell, 1996). This makes it difficult to consider pain *in itself* as an impairment or as a part of disability; additionally, there has been a great deal of work done by disabled people to distance themselves from medicine and the medicalization of disability. There is sometimes an attitude within disabled communities that wanting medical assistance or treatment (or even a cure for others in the future, if not for oneself (Wendell, 1996)[2] is the same as accepting the medical model (Kafer, 2013) and its many issues – there is no space left for the complexities of chronic illness.

As discussed in the first chapter, Tremain (2005) argues that discursive constructions of impairment within the social model reflect, maintain, and legitimize normality. Instead, if we consider that constructions of normal bodies and

DOI: 10.4324/9781003006237-3

somatic responses – and to follow this argument, pain is itself – are discursive productions, "cultural artefact[s] … in need of interpretation" (Best, 2007: 168), we can come to see that the body itself is socially constructed – that how we define and understand 'the body' is impacted and altered by social meanings and understandings. Thus impairment is "both an experience and a discursive construction" (Hughes and Paterson, 1997: 329), and there is a "need to construct an analysis of impairment that assumes our somatic sensations, including pain, are discursively constructed" (Best, 2007: 163). This is in contrast to understandings that position pain as inexpressible and beyond language (Langdridge and Butt, 2004; Scarry, 1985); somatic sensations are assumed to be outside of linguistic constraint or understanding, and thus beyond discursive construction.

This framing of pain as discursive construct may go some way to explaining why chronic pain and chronic illness have been objected to as impairments resulting in disablement/disability by proponents of the social model. Oliver (1996, 2013) has argued that because pain is universal and everyone, non-disabled and disabled alike, experiences pain at some point, pain is not a disability, but a medical problem alone.[3] In this view, pain is in effect *too normal* – too much a part of normal life – to be considered an impairment. For de Wolfe (2002), critiquing this viewpoint, pain is an 'embarrassment' that disability rights activists and some disability studies academics do not always want to engage with, and therefore "this reluctance relegates to the realm of the private, both conceptually and materially, those whose suffering cannot be relieved by either medical intervention or social change" (ibid., 2002: 255–256). While de Wolfe's equation of pain with suffering is problematic,[4] the argument instead demonstrates that a purely interactionist social model view of disability silences and isolates experiences of chronic illness and chronic pain.

Chronic illness, like chronic pain, is difficult to unpick into impairment and disability using a social model understanding, partly because of how illness is so firmly rooted in medicine, even more so than other conceptions of disability, and partly because chronic illness is understood as an individual – rather than a collective – experience, perhaps even an individual failure of self-control and self-regulation (we'll come to control in Chapters 5 and 6). Having already said that pain is discursive, I want to nonetheless recognize that chronic pain is difficult to grasp in terms of social construction, because, as Morris (1992) and Wendell (1996) have both pointed out, disability thus comes in when it comes to how normal concepts of time, function, and sensation are constructed, and it becomes much harder to distinguish between embodied impairment effects and the impact of social attitudes and barriers – in effect it is hard to draw a clear demarking line between impairment effects and social attitudes.

Pain is also largely ignored by those disability rights activists and disability studies academics who focus solely on disability as a positive identity – I would suggest this is partly due to the discomfort and 'embarrassment' de Wolfe (2002) discusses – and can thus tend toward side-lining research and activist engagement with vulnerability, fatigue, and pain. This problematic viewpoint is neatly encapsulated by Siebers, writing that:

> Physical pain is highly individualistic, unpredictable, and raw as reality. It pits the mind against the body in ways that makes the opposition between thought and ideology in most current body theory seem trivial. It offers few resources for resisting ideological constructions of masculinity and femininity, the erotic monopoly of the genitals, the violence of the ego, or the power of capital. Pain is not a friend to humanity. It is not a secret resource for political change. It is not a well of delight for the individual. Theories that encourage these interpretations are not only unrealistic about pain; they contribute to an ideology of ability that marginalizes people with disabilities and makes their stories of suffering and victimisation both politically impotent and difficult to believe.
>
> (Siebers, 2006: 178)

Of course, I both agree and disagree with Siebers – while pain is highly individualistic, it is also socially constructed; pain does exactly what he says it does not, in that pain can be a delight for the individual, and as BDSM practitioners have demonstrated, it can be a part of resisting power structures and exploring eroticism and pleasure beyond genital contact. Nonetheless, Siebers' view is typical of the issues that disability studies and activism has had with pain, situating it as *too individual* for activism or theory to properly address. I would contest that exploring how pain is socially constructed as well as experienced reveals much that resists and challenges ableism, offering a critique of the understanding of pain as always exclusively negative.

Whether from a social, positive, or medical model perspective, pain is positioned as pathological, as a deviance from norms (Best, 2007), especially when it continues over an abnormal length of time and thus becomes labeled as 'chronic pain.' However, in exploring embodied experiences of pain, we can note parallels between experiences of people living with chronic pain and those disabled people whose embodied experience is closer to the social model construction, with a fixed, known, and medically-recognized disability which is visible/noticeable to strangers. Chronic pain without an identifiable cause has no "culturally conditioned, straightforward label, as is available for many other health states, [which contributes] to … being alternatively, if not explicitly, labeled as somehow different or difficult" (Nielsen and Fernandez, 2010: 45). This labeling is a familiar one to disabled people, often given such labels when requesting reasonable adjustments or calling for greater attention to be given to their rights and/or needs.

Further parallels come about through a lack of social recognition, and a need to constantly 'prove' one's disability. For those living with chronic pain and/or illness, this can often start before a formal medical diagnosis is acquired (if diagnosis happens at all); diagnosis is used to gatekeep access to assistance or support, and thus living without a diagnosis can often be experienced as disabling specifically because it leaves one without access to the validation, knowledge, and support that comes in the form of community groups and spaces of shared experience. Invisible disabilities – ones requiring no obvious continually-used aid, or that do not visibly mark the body as somehow 'abnormal' – and undocumented disabilities (see Mollow, 2014) are often assumed to be non-existent; like disabled people with invisible disabilities, people living with chronic pain and illness must somehow 'prove' their disability (Richardson, 2005), not just for access to medical care, but also for social recognition. Patsavas draws attention to medics who identify 'risk factors' of chronic pain that "read more like character flaws than biological markers" (Patsavas, 2014: 210); the conflation of illness and disability with the moral state of a 'sufferer' is firmly embedded in culture.

The lack of social recognition – of being seen as being in pain – is further reflected in a lack of cultural resources for understanding or organizing experiences of chronic pain (Bendelow and Williams, 1995; Nielsen and Fernandez, 2010). This lack of understanding – and the hostility and confusion that it leads to – is often expressed as a social pressure not to talk about chronic pain, particularly for women, with the gendered discourse of the whining, weak, hysterical woman playing a key part in this silencing:

> This pressure may be exacerbated for women in cultures which admire the 'restitution narrative' (Frank, 1995) in which people are ill, recover, and 'return to normal', or in which certain illnesses are seen as discrediting and hence to be hidden … Cultural perceptions that women have a greater resilience to pain on a 'day-to-day' basis leads to the idea that women's pain does not therefore need to be taken seriously (Bendelow, 1993). Women therefore face a dual dilemma that expression of their pain is necessary if they want to be taken seriously, but, at the same time, this remains socially undesirable.
>
> (Richardson, 2005: 37)

This parallels with the experience of disabled people, who have not returned to, or have never been, 'normal,' and whose experiences are only rarely represented.

People living with chronic pain are often isolated (de Wolfe, 2002; Nielsen and Fernandez, 2010), partly through a lack of understanding from others (Morris, 1991), and even more so as a result of this ongoing pressure toward silence (Richardson, 2005), particularly in cultures where illness and disability are constructed as private experiences for the individual, not suitable to be seen or expressed in public (Wendell, 1996). Wendell observes that

> the inclination to keep those who are more than temporarily ill out of the stream of work and social activity is based as much on ignorance and prejudice as is the inclination to keep other people with disabilities hidden in the private realm.
>
> (ibid., 1996: 20)

Addressing disability with a more crip approach creates space within disability for chronic pain and chronic illness, arguing that the issue of "dividing experience into segments, of denying its fluidity, and of specifying a stable disabled identity … [is unworkable when] disabled people allude to a complex existence that occupies the space between health and illness, disability and normality" (de Wolfe, 2002: 258).

Cripping Pain?

In the first chapter, I discussed normative pain discourses; briefly, people who do not live with chronic pain regard being in pain as dehumanizing (Patsavas, 2014; Sheppard, 2014), as ontologically intolerable, if not ontologically impossible, and that those who do live with chronic pain exist solely and continually in a place of suffering. "The cultural discourses that frame pain as an isolating, devastating experience crystallize to prevent the exploration of alternative explanations for why chronic pain might be (or seem to be) unliveable" (Patsavas, 2014: 204); those who regard pain as other than wholly intolerable are regarded as perverse (Newmahr, 2011; Patsavas, 2014), or, more commonly, assumed to be lying about being in pain (Nielsen and Fernandez, 2010). The assumption that being in pain is intolerable, and reduces the person in pain down to an inhuman, animalistic, sufferer means that when people in pain present as anything other than inhuman they are disbelieved, even though presenting as inhuman means they are stigmatized and made abject. This discourse presents very little space for alternatives, or even for complexity in how chronic pain is lived with, while participants' narratives revealed a much more complicated experience.

From the outset, it is important to note that in arguing that the discourse of pain is restrictive and reductive, I do not intend to deny that the experience of chronic pain is not, and cannot be, devastating and difficult. I would instead argue as Patsavas does, "that when cultural discourses construct pain as the cause of feelings of devastation, they oversimplify complex cultural, historical, and political phenomena. More than that, they prevent us from examining the structural conditions that make experiences of chronic pain tragic" (2014: 204). This means that while chronic pain experiences can be devastating, the sensation of pain alone is not the *sole* cause of that devastation – there are structural conditions that mean living with chronic pain can be devastating. The abjection of people who speak of their chronic pain, and the assumption that chronic pain makes one inhuman are important structural conditions affecting how people living with chronic pain experience their pain – as are the structures of pace of life, and the demands of appropriate self-control. Analgesic culture relies on a discourse of pain as meaningless and devastating to support the push toward eliminating pain, and structural forces that support living with chronic pain as devastating – and prevent alternative narratives from being heard – do just that.

Bendelow and Williams (1995) viewed chronic pain as needing a *cause* or reason in order to prevent those living with it to experience despair and isolation. I would contend that it is the dismissal of chronic pain that leads to isolation, as Thomas and Johnson (2000) observe – rather than solely the pain itself. For some people with chronic pain, the lack of visible cause for their pain combines with the duration of the pain, leading to a sense of delegitimization, of feeling like the fakers and malingerers social discourses paints us (Richardson, 2005) – and expressing pain or fatigue to others can exacerbate this, while "the omnipresent nature of chronic pain created and continually [reinforces] a sense of isolation and estrangement from society" (Nielsen and Fernandez, 2010: 47) precisely because of the discourse that our pain cannot be understood by others. The assumption of devastation, in addition, increases this sense of delegitimization; in not being wholly and continuously devastated by pain – in not fitting the discursive expectation – we are assumed to not be in pain.

This assumption that chronic pain is not understandable – or that it is not real – makes it difficult for people living with chronic pain to discuss their experiences, especially when their experiences run counter to the narrative of what is "normal" or "supposed to be." In particular, there is difficulty in both living with pain *and* resisting narratives which position them as objects of pity and/or disbelief. Chronic pain means that pain becomes an everyday experience, a part of the self. One of my participants put it best, showing a deep awareness of how living with chronic pain had changed their phenomenological self;

> *If somebody asks me how I am, and I say, 'Oh well, I'm in a lot of pain,' but, you know, that would be the same answer every day. It's just, like, where does that go? It doesn't go anywhere, and… stuff like that. So, it becomes a norm as well. So it becomes something that is part of the norm that isn't spoken about as news because it's part of the norm, and a lot of other people forget that's your norm.*
>
> (Charlie, interview 2)

This new norm, being in pain, is the phenomenological self remade with pain. Just as new pain makes us aware of the body (Scarry, 1985; Young, 1997), once that awareness has 'settled in' to being a part of the everyday experience of the body, we cease to consider it as relevant – it does not erase other subjectivities of the self – and it is only when chronic pain changes that we become particularly aware of it once more. Rather than a remaking of the self *after* pain as occurs after acute pain, chronic pain's ongoing experience – with no expectation of ending – means that the self is remade *with* chronic pain – although writing it thus makes the experience seem rather straightforward. In exploring participants' narratives of sensation, I have explored how they have actively – and not so actively – remade themselves, and come to live with pain; in making chronic pain part of their lives, they crip pain.

Cure

Circling back to medical discourses which influence everyday discourse (as discussed in the earlier chapter), both acute and chronic pain are understood as signifying illness or injury. There is an assumption that there is a straight line from the symptoms of illness, to diagnosis, to cure (Snyder, 2004). This discourse of a stepwise, problem-solving approach has filtered from medicine to wider social discourses – we go to the doctor when we are ill, and we expect to be told what is wrong with us (even when we think we know beforehand), and we will receive a cure. This ties to what Frank (1995) calls the 'restitution narrative' – once the diagnosis and subsequent cure are received from the proper authorities, we 'get better', and return to normal once again, having been healed by whatever pill or potion the doctor has prescribed. In this discourse, as through much of the psychological and medical discourses, there is a conflation of cure and healing (Barker and Langdridge, 2009); this conflation extends into discourses around long-term or chronic illness, and disability; all of which are positioned as requiring *curing*, as problems to be solved. To start looking at chronic pain through a crip lens, it is important to consider what this positioning – and the expectation that an illness will be cured – does in terms of how chronic illness is understood (or misunderstood), and this requires a certain amount of unpicking of what is understood as *normal* within this discourse.

Particularly following an injury (this injury is usually assumed to be physical, although there are similar discourses of mental injury following traumatic events, such as bereavement), we go through a period of healing – it is this process of healing that 'cures' us; the most familiar might be being told to 'keep your weight off it for a few days' following a twisted ankle, or physiotherapy following a broken bone. Once this healing period is over, the cure is complete and we are 'normal' again; the more traumatic the injury, the longer the healing period – but this period must have an ending. In some cases, we go through part, or all, of this healing period under the care and gaze of professional rehabilitators – doctors, physiotherapists, nurses, and careworkers. The length of the healing period can be predicted – and prescribed – by these professionals; for a painful injury, the prediction of a particular length of time reassures the person that their pain will end, and reassures them that normality will be regained.

For many, this medicalized period of healing time can be experienced as a loss – a loss of self-control and self-knowledge, of power over your own body (Jain, 2013; Young, 1997); replaced by the power and knowledge of medical professionals and care workers, on whom the newly injured person may be dependent in ways they had not previously considered possible for themselves to become – a part of the broad failure of imagination when it comes to disability, Medical personnel can control how much input patients have over the rehabilitation period (even more so if it takes place in a hospital or other care setting), with a 'doctor knows best' attitude prevalent, especially when it comes to setting and achieving 'recovery milestones' (Sullivan, 2005) – but also in the diagnosis and prescription of cure. While pain can be – and frequently is – a part of this rehabilitation and healing process, the cessation of pain is expected once the process is over, and once the injured body is rehabilitated. In effect, pain is a sign that healing is incomplete.

This rehabilitation and healing process is conceptualized by Turner as a rebuilding process:

> [involving a] refashioning [of] the self. This remaking is not merely a discursive process; it involves, following Merleau-Ponty, the reconstruction of the lived, sensual body… [It] also takes place within the professional 'gaze' of rehabilitation which holds out the typically false promise of normalization, that is, the production of a socially 'normal' body – young, athletic, and sexual. It is not enough to return to society via rehabilitation; the rehabilitated body has to be discursively normal.
>
> (Turner, 2001: 258)

in order to be fully cured. It is interesting to note here that Turner doesn't even mention being pain-free as a condition of normality; being pain-free is such a key part of having a normal body that it is immediately assumed that the two are one and the same; being without pain is rendered invisible by its very position as normal. This process of achieving normality, at least as far as the body is concerned, is also about rendering the body docile to systems of power and government (Sullivan, 2005) and once again capable of productive work within capitalism. The body in pain is not a docile body, but at least it does not disturb others, unless the body speaks and the experience of pain is expressed; because the body-not-in-pain is so normal, so invisible, bodies are assumed to be bodies-not-in-pain until they are revealed as otherwise, especially when those bodies have no other outward signifiers of disability. Through shaming and stigma people who live with chronic pain learn not to talk of their pain, to become outwardly docile-normal bodies, to be civilized and self-controlled.

Shaming and stigma – and access to medical care – is not equally distributed. Access to medical care is unequal (both in the UK, and globally); not all the participants felt they had access to adequate medical care, particularly when it came to being seen by chronic pain specialists. This unequal access can be geographic – not living near a specialist – as well as financial; like myself, all the participants accessed their medical care tied to chronic pain through the NHS, which has its own peculiarities and intricacies, not least in terms of what is available in the local area[5] and what is an acceptable treatment.[6]

Unequal access also lies in discrimination and the perceptions of carers and medics; just as women and people of color are less likely to be believed when reporting care (Bendelow, 1993; Hoffman et al., 2016; Hoffman and Tarzian, 2001; Trawalter et al., 2014), gender and sexual minorities are less likely to receive adequate care (Jain, 2013), or face discrimination (Earle, 1999), as are fat people (Gordon, 2020; Hobbes, 2018). As Jain observes, people "who have experienced, or interpreted, discrimination are less likely to visit doctors for check-ups or to follow up on health concerns" (2013: 39), and this then leads to additional problems, such as illnesses not being diagnosed until later stages and a lack of necessary medication. Medical care is not free of value judgments. For Charlie, access to care is complicated not just by being trans, but by being autistic, as they explain;

> *I find it difficult to sometimes be taken seriously or get the support or care I need sometimes by that, because I don't express my pain in ways that are socially the norm.*
> (Charlie, interview 2)

The pressure to express pain appropriately and, when pain is expressed, the resulting stigma of failing to contain pain (Nielsen and Fernandez, 2010) leads to inadequate care when medics act as gatekeepers to specialist care, as well as acting as care providers themselves. Thus, people living with chronic pain negotiate an unequal system in different ways, depending on the stigma they experience – which will vary depending on a range of factors beyond their control.

This stigmatizing of people with chronic pain comes, in part, from the discourse of health and risk; this discourse creates a victim-blaming approach to illness, placing the onus for not preventing their illness – or dealing with it in the 'correct' way – on the ill person. People who are perceived as having done something to cause, or not done something to prevent their illness, are treated less sympathetically, and stigmatized (Bendelow, 2006) – by medical professionals, carers, other people, and even other people with the self-same illness or impairment; we see this distinctly when looking at the experiences of fat people in the healthcare system (Gordon, 2020; Hobbes, 2018). Discussing pain specifically, Richardson observes that "as members of a society which shares a cultural understanding of pain, sufferers may be both the subjects of, and makers of, 'misguided inferences' about pain and its legitimacy" (2005: 36). This stigma is gendered and racialized; women with chronic pain report feeling greater stigma, and being taken less seriously when they seek medical help (Bendelow, 1993; Hoffman and Tarzian, 2001). Bendelow (1993) considers that this may well be tied to the societal belief that women tolerate pain better – they have 'higher pain thresholds' – but that they 'give in' more easily to pain than men, who are able to 'push through it.' For women of color, this effect is added to by the perception – rooted in 18th and 19th century 'scientific' discourse that dehumanized non-white people, women, and children (Morris, 1991) – that black and brown bodies are 'less sensitive' to pain, and black women, in particular, are more able to cope with high levels of pain without help (Hoffman et al., 2016; Staton et al., 2007; Trawalter et al., 2014). This is echoed in discourses positioning black athletes as less civilized and more animal-like than their white counterparts (Trawalter et al., 2014), less sensitive to pain and more capable of 'powering through.'

The acquisition of a diagnosis may open the doors to particular forms of recognition and support, but can also act as a further stigma. For Julie and Michelle, their diagnoses were experienced as limiting their access to care – they both felt that once they had been given diagnoses, that was it, they were on their own, because no 'cure' could be given, and they had no prospect of 'improvement' or successful rehabilitation. Both Julie and Michelle – and also Charlie and Rita, to lesser degrees – experienced what Bury refers to as a 'crisis of credibility,' which "may occur if the individual continues to report problems after their 'share' of attention has been used up, or when they have been placed in a category (e.g., 'successful operation') which closes off avenues of support and information" (Bury, 1991: 457). The acquisition of a 'dustbin diagnosis' – a broad 'syndrome' rather than a specific illness, or a diagnosis for which no cure exists[7] is often experienced as a dismissal, especially as the diagnosis itself can take years of effort on the part of both medics and patients; medics' frustration with the lack of either clear causes and/or cure may spill over to frustration with patients, who are themselves frustrated with the same issue (Patsavas, 2014; Tomlinson, 2013; Wendell, 1996).

Cure and Stigma

For many disabled people 'cure' can be seen as an attempt to wipe out disabled people (and being disabled as an identity itself), coming from an ableist assumption that the deepest wish of disabled people is to be 'normal', to be able-bodyminded – together with the assumption that disabled people must be suffering, and their lives must be ontologically intolerable (Kumari Campbell, 2009). Wendell puts it best, for me, when she writes:

> I find that my own resistance to the attitude that I need to be 'cured' in order to be a whole or fully acceptable person infuses my desire for a 'cure' with ambivalence. I want to have more energy and less pain, and to have a more predictable body; about that there is no ambivalence. Moreover, I feel heart-sore when I hear about someone else being diagnosed with M.E.; how could I not want a cure for everyone else who suffers with it? Yet I cannot wish that I had never contracted M.E., because it has made me a different person, a person I am glad to be, would not want to have missed being, and could not imagine relinquishing, even if I were 'cured'.
>
> (1996: 83)

For myself, I see Wendell's wish for a cure for everyone else not as a need for just a simplistic cure, but as a need for ME/CFS to be understood – and recognized in terms of the experiences of those who have it – as well as for chronic illness to be recast as a source of knowledge; the acknowledgment that the lives of disabled people are worth living, before and without cure or rehabilitation.

The "moral dimension of beliefs and practices surrounding different health states" (Bury, 1991: 456) results in stigma experienced by people with chronic pain, as well as people with other diagnoses (Illich, 1995). Despite the figures of incidence of chronic pain, the medical approach to illness and disability universalizes experiences – expecting illness and disability to fit particular patterns of behavior and progress (Wendell, 1996) in the rehabilitation narrative discussed previously. For many like Michelle and Julie, the labels 'chronic fatigue', 'fibromyalgia', or simply 'chronic pain' can be seen as a sort of dustbin diagnosis – where the diagnosis is more often seen as an umbrella term (a 'syndrome' rather than an illness, as in *chronic fatigue syndrome*), a shorthand for 'we don't know what to do with you'; for participants in Nielsen and Fernandez's study into patient experiences, "the lack of a culturally condoned, straightforward label for their condition, as is available for many other health states, contributed to participants being alternatively, if not explicitly, labeled as somehow different or difficult" (2010: 45), with this stigma leading to under-treatment or dismissal (Patsavas, 2014; Wendell, 1996).

It is not just the patients' perceptions of their experiences that indicate this stigma; "in a study of 268 registered nurses, the chronic pain sufferer was negatively stereotyped and judged to have less intense suffering than an individual with acute pain" (Thomas and Johnson, 2000: 684). The stigmatization of people in chronic pain by medics and healthcare professionals can have very real effects, such as when Morris explains that:

> American doctors regularly refuse to prescribe effective doses of narcotic painkillers to dying patients [with terminal cancer] on the grounds that the

> patients might become addicted. The treatment of cancer pain, clearly, is still not based solely on scientific fact but draws on ignorance, fear, prejudice, and on an invisible, unacknowledged moral codes expressing half-baked notions about the evil of drugs and the duty to bear affliction.
>
> (Morris, 1991: 192)

The situation Morris describes have since come full circle; in the late 1990s through to the early 2010s, there was a greater willingness to prescribe painkillers, in particular to terminal cancer patients. However, more recently – at the time when this research was being conducted – there has since been a response to widespread opiate painkiller prescribing (particularly in the United States, but also in the UK) which has seen a reversal of this approach – including NICE guidance for the NHS recommending against painkiller prescribing for people living with chronic pain (NICE, 2021), with chronically pained people concerned as to how this will impact (and be impacted by) the stigma they experience as pained people.

This may seem at odds with my previous explanation that we live in an analgesic culture. However, as Patsavas explains, narratives of ending suffering and the dangers of opioid painkillers

> work together to bind the chronic pain 'sufferer' within a discursive system that offers a cure through consumption, condemns the individual for using that cure, and holds the individual responsible when the cure does not work. Living a life without pain amounts to an imperative that captures the person in pain within a system of individual responsibility and 'compulsory able-bodiedness'.
>
> (Patsavas, 2014: 209–210)

It is this, together with the idealizing of being pain-free which makes our culture analgesic; very literally, we wish to stop pain. Catherine mentioned that she felt that her doctors had recently become less willing – or less able, in that strictures have been imposed on them – to prescribe painkillers, which was affecting her wellbeing as well as her confidence in the care provided. This complex tangle of pressure to manage pain appropriately through medicine, to express pain appropriately, and to be rehabilitated or cured properly works within wider ableist discourses, limiting discussion of care to medicine, dismissing non-medical care, but also condemning the individual when medical care fails them.

The condemnation of those whose medical care has failed to rehabilitate/cure them spreads outside of the medical sphere, just as illness and incapacity affects multiple aspects of people's lives, including their relationships. As Julie wrote:

> *I can't just park my health problems to one side and enjoy sex/wank/kink/pain/whatever. They have to come too. And that's a big ask of others. Because nobody likes to think that their nudging to me to go for a third orgasm with an element of pain play involved results in a potential stroke.*
>
> (Julie, diary)

While Julie is talking specifically about uncommitted, non-monogamous relationships based around BDSM play, her words echo the discourse that tells disabled people that their disability makes them undesirable partners – especially if they require care or assistance (Gillespie-Sells et al., 1998; Shakespeare et al., 1996). The dual assumptions that disabled people require their intimate partners to also be carers,[8] and that care work is demeaning and disgusting whether it is paid or not, work against disabled people and also limits what is perceived of as care. Within these assumptions care consists of physical labor and wiping away bodily fluids, but not of slowing your walk to match a different pace, or sitting with a person experiencing a panic attack; being the object of care, being cared for, is positioned as demeaning or discomforting. Within this narrative care is not an act of love or of recognizing another's inherent human dignity[9] (Piepzna-Samarasinha, 2018) but an act that is demeaning toward both giver and receiver of care.

Price (2015) and Piepzna-Samarasinha (2018) illustrate reimaginings of care as collective which is focused on non-medical care, but when taken alongside Kafer's (2013) call for space for medicine within disability rights and crip spaces and calls to acknowledge the interdependence of life (Crow, 1996; Morris, 1992; Wendell, 1996), Price's description paints an arresting image of collective care which:

> *Means moving together and being limited together. It means giving more when one has the ability to do so, and accepting help when that is needed. It does not mean knowing exactly what another's pain feels like, but it does mean respecting each person's pain as real and important. Finally, care must emerge between subjects considered to be equally valuable (which does not necessarily mean that both are operating from similar places of rationality), and it must be participatory in nature, that is, developed through the desires and needs of all participants.*
>
> (Price, 2015: 279)

This reimagining of care has space for complexity, for acknowledging that disabled people can perform care for others. Natalie's description of her relationship with her partner, who is also disabled, comes close to Price's description; she trusts that her needs will be heard, and met – but also that her partner will express his needs, and trust her with those needs – and for them, this comes down to communicating their bodily states;

> *It's something we have to discuss a lot, because we're very tactile outside of love-making and we both have times when there's a part of our body we can't stand to have touched. Other times, there are parts that benefit greatly from touch, such as rubbing a cramping muscle etc... So, we talk about it all the time – not analytically, not in a self-pitying way, but we keep one another informed.*
>
> (Natalie, interview 1)

Conclusion

Cripping pain exposes the normative expectations and discourses of pain – in particular the expectation that chronic pain cannot be lived with, and that pain is unwanted. Being without pain is assumed as not just the default but the ideal, in much the same way as being able-bodyminded is. In the next chapter, I turn to how kink play also exposes and challenges discourses of pain.

Notes

1 See Introduction for their profiles.
2 We will get to cure shortly, I promise.
3 Oliver changed his mind.
4 And we'll get to that too.
5 for example, while undertaking this research project, I moved from one area of London to another, necessitating a change of GP, and unwittingly moved from one NHS Local Authority to another; the first routinely referred people with chronic pain to a specialist clinic, while the second did not – luckily this was picked up by the clinic, who moved me up the waiting list to ensure I was already under their care before I moved.
6 For chronic pain/illness (and particularly people living with ME/CFS, as well as fibromyalgia), the recommendation of Graded Exercise Therapy is decided by NICE.
7 Examples of such diagnoses include ME/CFS and fibromyalgia.
8 Which can of course be the case, but is neither universal nor wanted (even when necessary).
9 I recognize 'dignity' is itself a contentious topic (Frazee, 2014).

References

Barker M and Langdridge D (2009) Silencing Accounts of Silenced Sexualities. In: Ryan-Flood R and Gil R (eds) *Secrecy and Silence in the Research Process: Feminist Reflections*. Abingdon: Routledge, pp. 86–98.
Bendelow G (1993) Pain Perceptions, Emotions and Gender. *Sociology of Health and Illness* 15(3): 273–294. DOI: 10.1111/1467–9566.ep10490526.
Bendelow G (2006) Pain, Suffering and Risk. *Health, Risk and Society* 8(1): 59–70.
Bendelow G and Williams SJ (1995) Transcending the Dualisms: Towards a Sociology of Pain. *Sociology of Health and Illness* 17(2): 139–165.
Best S (2007) The Social Construction of Pain: An Evaluation. *Disability & Society* 22(2): 161–171. DOI: 10.1080/09687590601141592.
Bury M (1991) The Sociology of Chronic Illness: A Review of Research and Prospects. *Sociology of Health and Illness* 13(4): 451–468.
Crow L (1996) Including All Our Lives: Renewing the Social Model of Disability. In: Morris J (ed) *Encounters with Strangers: Feminism and Disability*. London: The Women's Press, pp. 55–73.
de Wolfe P (2002) Private Tragedy in Social Context? Reflections on Disability, Illness and Suffering. *Disability & Society* 17(3): 255–267.
Earle S (1999) Facilitated Sex and the Concept of Sexual Need: Disabled Students and Their Personal Assistants. *Disability & Society* 14(3): 309–323.
Frank AW (1995) *The Wounded Storyteller*. Chicago, IL: University of Chicago Press.
Frazee C (2014) There Can Be Dignity in All States of Life. *The Ottawa Citizen*, 14 October. Ottawa.
Gillespie-Sells K, Hill M and Robbins B (1998) *She Dances to Different Drums: Research into Disabled Women's Sexuality*. London: King's Fund.

Gordon A (2020) *What We Don't Talk about When We Talk about Fat*. Boston, MA: Beacon Press.

Hobbes M (2018) Everything You Know about Obesity Is Wrong. *Highline*. Available at: https://highline.huffingtonpost.com/articles/en/everything-you-know-about-obesity-is-wrong/.

Hoffman DE and Tarzian AJ (2001) The Girl Who Cried Pain: A Bias Against Women in the Treatment of Pain. *Journal of Law, Medicine and Ethics* 29(1): 13–27. DOI: 10.1111/j.1748-720X.2001.tb00037.x.

Hoffman KM, Trawalter S, Axt JR, et al. (2016) Racial Bias in Pain Assessment and Treatment Recommendations, and False Beliefs about Biological Differences Between Blacks and Whites. *Proceedings of the National Academy of Sciences of the United States of America* 113(16): 4296–4301. DOI: 10.1073/pnas.1516047113.

Hughes B and Paterson K (1997) The Social Model of Disability and the Disappearing Body: Towards a Sociology of Impairment. *Disability & Society* 12(3): 325–340. DOI: 10.1080/09687599727209.

Illich I (1995) *Limits to Medicine: Medical Nemesis, the Expropriation of Health*. London: Marion Boyars Publishers Ltd.

Jain SL (2013) *Malignant: How Cancer Becomes Us*. Oakland: University of California Press.

Kafer A (2013) *Feminist, Queer, Crip*. Bloomington and Indianapolis: Indiana University Press.

Kumari Campbell F (2009) *Contours of Ableism: The Production of Disability and Abledness*. Basingstoke: Palgrave Macmillan.

Langdridge D and Butt T (2004) A Hermeneutic Phenomenological Investigation of the Construction of Sadomasochistic Identities. *Sexualities* 7(1): 31–53. DOI: 10.1177/1363460704040137.

Mollow A (2014) Criphystemologies: What Disability Theory Needs to Know about Hysteria. *Journal of Literary & Cultural Disability Studies* 8(2): 185–201. DOI: 10.3828/jlcds.2014.15.

Morris DB (1991) *The Culture of Pain*. Berkeley: University of California Press.

Morris J (1992) Personal and Political: A Feminist Perspective on Researching Physical Disability. *Disability, Handicap & Society* 7(2): 157–166.

Newmahr S (2011) *Playing on the Edge: Sadomasochism, Risk, and Intimacy*. Bloomington: Indiana University Press.

NICE (2021) *Chronic Pain (Primary and Secondary) in Over 16s: Assessment of All Chronic Pain and Management of Chronic Primary Pain*. NG193, April. National Institute for Health and Care Excellence.

Nielsen A and Fernandez J (2010) Journeys with Chronic Pain: Acquiring Stigma along the Way. In: *Making Sense of Pain: Critical and Interdisciplinary Perspectives*. Oxford: Inter-Disciplinary Press, pp. 45–54.

Oliver M (1996) Defining Impairment and Disability: Issues at Stake. In: Barnes C and Mercer G (eds) *Exploring the Divide*. Leeds: The Disability Press, pp. 29–54.

Oliver M (2013) Distinctly Disabled. Available at: http://www.disabilitynow.org.uk/article/distinctly-disabled (accessed 29 September 2013).

Patsavas A (2014) Recovering a Cripistemology of Pain: Leaky Bodies, Connective Tissue, and Feeling Discourse. *Journal of Literary & Cultural Disability Studies* 8(2): 203–218. DOI: 10.3828/jlcds.2014.16.

Piepzna-Samarasinha LL (2018) *Care Work: Dreaming Disability Justice*. Vancouver: Arsenal Pulp Press.

Price M (2015) The Bodymind Problem and the Possibilities of Pain. *Hypatia* 30(1): 268–284. DOI: 10.1111/hypa.12127.

Richardson JC (2005) Establishing the (Extra)Ordinary in Chronic Widespread Pain. *Health: An Interdisciplinary Journal of the Social Study of Health, Illness and Medicine* 9(1): 31–48.

Scarry E (1985) *The Body in Pain: The Making and Unmaking of the World*. New York: Oxford University Press.

Seymour W (1998) *Remaking the Body: Rehabilitation and Change*. St Leonards: Unwin.

Shakespeare T, Gillespie-Sells K and Davies D (1996) *The Sexual Politics of Disability: Untold Desires*. London and New York: Cassell.

Sheppard E (2014) Crippling Pain: Examining Pain in Discourses of Normal Human Experience. In: *Theorising Normalcy and the Mundane: More Questions of the Human*. University of Sheffield.

Siebers T (2006) Disability in Theory: From Social Constructionism to the New Realism of the Body. In: Davies LJ (ed) *The Disability Studies Reader*. 2nd ed. Abingdon: Routledge, pp. 173–183.

Snyder CR (2004) Physical Pain ≠ Suffering: A Personal Commentary on Coping. *International Perspectives on Stress and Coping* 10(1): 51–71.

Staton LJ, Panda M, Chen I, et al. (2007) When Race Matters: Disagreement in Pain Perception Between Patients and Their Physicians in Primary Care. *Journal of the National Medical Association* 99(5): 532–538.

Sullivan M (2005) Paraplegia, Rehabilitation, and the Politics of Movement. In: Tremain S (ed) *Foucault and the Government of Disability*. Ann Arbo: University of Michigan Press, pp. 27–44.

Thomas SP and Johnson M (2000) A Phenomenologic Study of Chronic Pain. *Western Journal of Nursing Research* 22(6): 683–705.

Tomlinson J (2013) How Doctors Respond to Chronic Pain. In: *A Better NHS: Exploring the Relationships Between Doctors and Patients and Health Policy*. Available at: https://abetternhs.wordpress.com/2013/09/07/pain/ (accessed 1 July 2016).

Trawalter S, Hoffman KM and Waytz A (2014) Racial Bias in Perceptions of Others' Pain. *PLoS ONE* 11(3). DOI: 10.1371/journal.pone.0152334.

Tremain S (2005) Foucault, Governmentality, and Critical Disability Theory. In: Tremain S (ed) *Foucault and the Government of Disability*. Ann Arbor: University of Michigan Press, pp. 1–24.

Turner BS (2001) Disability and the Sociology of the Body. In: Albrecht GL, Seelman KD and Bury M (eds) *Handbook of Disability Studies*. London: Sage, pp. 252–267.

Wendell S (1996) *The Rejected Body: Feminist Philosophical Reflections on Disability*. New York: Routledge.

Young K (1997) *Presence in the Flesh: The Body in Medicine*. Cambridge, MA: Harvard University Press.

3 Add BDSM, Stir

BDSM stands for bondage and discipline, dominance and submission, sadism and masochism (Bauer, 2014; Langdridge and Barker, 2007; Taylor and Ussher, 2001); while this is a fairly broad umbrella term, it does not necessarily leave room for everything which could come into the participants' practices in which they experience pain. I have therefore chosen to use *kink* as the umbrella term, although I use BDSM a lot as well. As discussed previously, this is both a wider range of practices and preferences, as well as the term participants generally used themselves – they described themselves as *kinky* and what they did as *kink* or *play*.[1] This chapter will look at disability and sex, somewhat briefly – to give context for the discussion of BDSM/kink. And then, once again, I will bring in my participants' words and experiences, digging into their kink pain.

Disability, Sex, and BDSM

When I talk about this project, I sometimes like to tell the story of getting it through the ethics committee; the project was reviewed and eventually passed, after some wrangling, as a committee member felt that while my approach considered the ethics carefully and went beyond the standards expected by the university, they found the topic *itself* problematic. They considered asking disabled people to discuss BDSM practices rather discomforting, and wondered if it might be seen as encouraging vulnerable people to take part in dangerous practices they did not have the capacity to consent to. This, to me, highlighted rather starkly the asexualization and infantilization of disabled people that is particularly notable when it comes to sex and sexuality,[2] especially in conjunction with non-normative practices and/or sexualities. In discussing how chronic pain and kink fit together and what they tell us about the other, the asexualization[3] of disabled people is a significant discourse; there is the assumption that, on becoming disabled, a person swaps sexuality and sexual activity for disablement – and this includes becoming chronically ill and/or pained. For some who live with chronic pain, sexual dysfunction can be a problem – either as a whole or part of their impairment, but, as Verschuren et al point out, "sexual dysfunction as a side effect of chronic disease has long been ignored in both research and clinical practice"

DOI: 10.4324/9781003006237-4

(Verschuren et al., 2010: 153), and such research and practice that there is overwhelmingly focuses on erectile dysfunction or reproductive problems, essentializing sex to hetero-normative practices and reproductive capacity. So let us spend some time with disability and sexuality, before looking at BDSM.

The approaches to disabled people's sexuality can be broadly divided into two camps: reproduction and asexualization. Both are medicalized discourses that objectify disabled people, frequently with the "viewpoint of regulating the fertility of the dangerous female, as well as assisting the damaged male to regain his potency" (Waxman Fiduccia, 2000: 168). The medical model defines disability in terms of lack, and when it comes to sex and sexuality, there is an assumption of abnormality (Shakespeare et al., 1996), and problems – either disabled people have problems with their sex lives, or their sex lives and sexualities are problems in themselves. Thus, disabled people's sexuality is always abnormal.

This abnormality is also because, to quote Shildrick, "even when disabled people are sexually conservative in their own identities, their active sexual expression – if they have one – may necessarily fall outside of heteronormativity" (2009: 60). Hetero-normativity is not a particularly wide-ranging grouping, with sex for pleasure in particular being only hetero-normative when the – preferably monogamous – couple are white, heterosexual, able-bodyminded, young, and conventionally attractive (Tepper, 2000), and having sex that rarely strays beyond the 'vanilla.'[4] Arguments can of course be made that this reading of hetero-normativity as white, able, young, and conventionally attractive (and middle class, healthy, and monogamous) excludes most people from hetero-normativity in some way – but if instead it functions as an ideal, this regulation of sexual activity serves to exclude most those who are furthest from the ideal.

The abnormal disabled person whose sexuality or sexual activity is a problem is one who expresses that sexuality, and sexual desire, with a body that 'should not' be sexual – one that should not be desirable to others, or capable of reproducing a potentially disabled future (Kafer, 2013). This fear of disabled people's reproductive capabilities is heavily gendered, in that it tends to be disabled women's reproductive capabilities (and sexualities) that are most feared, and also most medicalized. However, this discourse is also impacted by the 'type' of impairment; people with learning disabilities and those with congenital impairments and 'severe' disabilities are more likely to be cast as in need of fertility control, as "although overtly eugenic excesses are relatively uncommon in the contemporary West, the psychic discomfort provoked by manifest differences that undermine cultural normativities is still operative" (Shildrick, 2009: 56). Disabled people are "not viewed as acceptable candidates for reproduction or even capable of sex for pleasure. We are viewed as childlike and in need of protection" (Tepper, 2000: 285). Thus the disabled body is cast as permanently dependent and childlike, and preferably kept that way through medical intervention (Kafer, 2013) or through the enforcement of 'protective' structures that can act instead as a removal of choice and personal power. Disabled children frequently receive little to no sex education, particularly if educated at segregated (or 'specialist') schools, and there is an expectation that disabled children will not become sexually active adults (Bahner, 2021; Shakespeare et al., 1996), with information withheld in order not to 'confuse' them, or 'encourage' sexual activity (Rogers, 2009).[5]

For disabled adults of any gender there is the assumption that physical impairment results in a complete lack of sexual or reproductive function, and therefore a lack of sexual desire (Shakespeare et al., 1996) and a lack of sexuality itself (Shildrick, 2009). When disabled people are imagined as sexually active, it is frequently thought that they will only have sex with other disabled people (Crossan and Monaghan, 2013; Liddiard, 2019; Shakespeare et al., 1996); disabled people are the only people who should find other disabled people sexually desirable. The positioning of disabled people as childlike and vulnerable further aids in this perception; desiring the/a disabled body is stigmatized and suspect (Kumari Campbell, 2009; Waxman Fiduccia, 2000), with the able person cast as predatory, even pedophilic, preying on vulnerable, innocent, childlike disabled people. For devotees, those who have a sexual or fetishistic attraction to people with specific impairments,[6] besides being cast as predatory[7] (Aguilera, 2000; Kafer, 2013; Solvang, 2007) and exploiting vulnerable disabled people, having their sexual attraction cast as a fetish means that, "reading between the lines, the implication … is that someone who would actually be attracted to a person with a disability must be sick" (Aguilera, 2000: 258).

For disabled cis women, "sexist stereotypes of women reinforce prejudices about disability …. in both cases, dependency, vulnerability, and frailty are the dominant association in patriarchal culture" (Shakespeare et al., 1996: 59). This gendered discourse of disability places disabled women as in need of protection – presumably from predatory violence, but also from their own inherently dangerous biology, as the case of Ashley X so clearly demonstrates (Kafer, 2013); disabled women's bodies are marked as dangerous if they are not forced to be asexual and non-reproductive. For women with acquired disabilities, this can cause conflict in relationships, as anecdata and "evidence suggests that, in heterosexual contexts, disabled men are more likely to maintain their relationships, while disabled women are more likely to find themselves abandoned by their erstwhile partner" (Shakespeare et al., 1996: 95). This is undoubtedly tied to "discourses of women with disabilities as non-gendered, non-sexual, childlike and dependent … [and therefore] unable to be sexual, spouses, partners or mothers" (Zitzelsberger, 2005: 395–396).

For disabled cis men, "popular notions of disabled masculinity focus obsessively on perceived impotence and lack of manhood" (Shakespeare et al., 1996: 97), and in the case of acquired disability, a loss of normative bodily function – particularly when it comes to the ability to get and sustain an erection – is often assumed to be accompanied by a loss of desire for sexual intimacy (Shildrick, 2009). Disability is positioned as a loss of masculinity, with Shakespeare et al. (1996) arguing that for many physically disabled men, masculinity must be either adapted or rejected. The "inability to perform gender and sexuality in a way that meets dominant societal expectations is seen as an intrinsic limitation, an 'unfortunate' but unavoidable consequence of inhabiting a disabled body" (Rembis, 2010: 51), particularly within a medical/tragedy model viewpoint; the standards of hetero-normative masculine behavior cannot be performed by a body that fails to meet the standards of hetero-normative ableism.[8] For some men, disability can also act as a 'release' from the demands of fulfilling a masculine gender role (Shakespeare et al., 1996), with the presumed inadequacy of deviation from the norm (Tepper, 2000) acting instead as 'permission' to explore beyond heteronormative ideals of masculine sexual behavior – which some disabled men feels gives them an advantage over non-disabled men in terms of their willingness – and enthusiastic participation – to engage in sexual practices beyond penis-in-vagina sex (Guldin, 2000).

The focus on reproductive potential in medicine (as well as wider systemic heterosexism) means that LGBTQ+ people are ignored and made invisible; they are frequently not mentioned by medical studies – less than 1% of public health studies are explicitly about LGBTQ+ people (Boehmer, 2002) – with the majority of those focused on HIV/AIDs (Boehmer, 2002; Branstrom and van der Star, 2013; Coulter et al., 2014). LGBTQ+ populations are excluded from concerns around fertility and reproduction, and, like disabled people, there is the "suspicion by majority populations that they cannot, will not, or should not contribute to the future of the human race. They will not reproduce, but if they do, the expectation is that the results will be tainted" (Siebers, 2012: 41). This 'reproductive irrelevance' means that there is little discussion of LGBTQ+ disabled people's sexuality or sex lives, beyond aspects around education and control, where their sexuality is once again positioned as a problem.

Disability studies itself has been accused of a heterosexual and hetero-normative bias when it comes to sexuality, and of continuing to use binary concepts of gender, sex, and sexuality (Tremain, 2000), treating gender, sex, and sexuality as fixed and natural, rather than sociocultural constructs – this is particularly apparent in aspects of the discipline that assume a medical model position. Greenwell and Hough's meta-study (2008) of articles with keywords or titles including both 'disability' and 'sex,' published between 2002 and 2006 showed that while 84 articles were published, only two mentioned trans as a gender variant, while three-quarters did not include data on sexual orientation of any participants. More recently, McRuer and Mollow (2012) write that the attention paid to non-hetero-normative disabled people has grown – and as crip theory approaches gain popularity, will continue to grow[9] – but research into disability and sexuality remains a niche area, and there is a continued need to move beyond binaries and tolerance (Rembis, 2010).

Lastly, another aspect of the infantilization of disabled people and the hetero-normative bias in Disability Studies that needs mentioning is how both of these have interacted with and reinforced cis-normativity and transphobia, especially in recent years. This isn't something I originally planned to discuss in the project – and something that has really only become more apparent in the years since the fieldwork itself was completed – but also something I cannot ignore. In part this is because of the participants themselves; there were four who are autistic, and their experiences as autistic people with chronic pain became part of the discussion – a higher than expected number, although there is evidence that autistic people are more likely to have multiple disabilities and chronic illnesses (Treating Autism et al., 2014). But just as importantly, I cannot ignore this because I believe – as a cis, queer, disabled woman – that trans and disabled solidarity is crucial to the survival of all our communities (see Goodley et al., 2019). Essentially, the positioning of disabled people as vulnerable to abuse and exploitation (and there is plenty of evidence that disabled people do experience more violence in their lives, including sexual assault, rape, and domestic violence (Gillespie-Sells et al., 1998; Mailhot Amborski et al., 2022; Office for National Statistics, 2019)) and their infantilization, particularly the infantilization of autistic young people and adults, is used as part of the discourse that trans, non-binary, and gender non-conforming autistic people are being deliberately exploited by 'trans activists' (a dog whistle term); that trans people exploit autistic people because their autism makes them more vulnerable. This plays into the positioning of people whose gender and/or sexual identities are non-normative as *perverted* – it is the same positioning that gay men are pedophiles, and the same moral panic over gay and lesbian young people that was seen in the 1980s.

BDSM and Kink

Speaking of perverted, let's turn now to BDSM.[10] BDSM (or kink) is also largely understood in normative discourses as about sex and the erotic, "despite recognition that SM is not always considered sex by participants … [with] some SM participants [rejecting] a sexual context for their S&M participation" (Newmahr, 2011: 66). This is not tidy delineation however; there is a great deal of variation across BDSM communities as to the level in which BDSM involves sex or sexuality, including a discussion of whether 'kinky' is in itself a sexual identity rather than a series of bodily practices. The difference between the two is largely split along the lines of whether or not a person who engages in BDSM is doing so as a form of bodily practice – erotic or not – but does not identify those practices as a key aspect of their selves, and is instead engaging with BDSM in the same way as they engage with hobbies; those hobbies may be looked down on or stigmatized, but the self is not. This sounds much simpler than it is in lived reality. On the other side are those for whom BDSM is a key aspect of their sexual selves, defining who they are attracted to, have sex with, and how they go about having sex – and thus it impacts on their wider social identities in the same way as being gay or asexual, and as such can be considered a minority identity in receipt of stigma; it is the self that is stigmatized.

Divisions within kink communities occur along multiple lines; tensions exist along these lines and within communities, and normative constructions cannot be considered as fixed. Beyond the identity/practice divide, divisions occur along the lines of geographical location, of sexuality and gender, of preferences for particular activities, and between 'old guard' and 'new guard' – and just to complicate things, where the line between old and new guards is drawn. Weiss defines the old guard as members of the primarily homosexual leather scene between the 1950s and 1970s, while from the 1980s onwards, the new guard – or new school – are pansexual, and less concentrated in urban centers (Bauer, 2007; Weiss, 2011). Rubin (1998) separates the new and old guards along degrees of in/formality, adherence to particular forms of etiquette, and the learning of skills rather than training; like Weiss, Rubin locates the old guard in the homosexual leather scene. Baldwin (1991) explains that the old guard's focus on ritual and formal rules originates in the large numbers of scene members in the 1950s onwards who were also military ex-servicemen, due to conscription and national service; while Baldwin is primarily discussing the West coast of the USA (particularly San Francisco), the influence of military and biker cultures on the leather scene in the UK and Europe is quickly apparent in the aesthetics.[11] The new guard, being less formal or rule-focused (and, justifiably, less concerned about the risks of a wider and more open membership following the legalization of homosexuality, although BDSM involvement still carries a stigma (Beckmann, 2014; Kleinplatz and Moser, 2006; Langdridge and Barker, 2007; Newmahr, 2011; Taylor and Ussher, 2001; Weiss, 2011)), is less easily identifiable than the old guard; as Bauer explains:

> the social organization of the Old Guard has mostly been replaced by a community that is open to anyone interested in joining, that educates its members through handbooks [rather than a system of training and 'apprenticeships'], workshops and so on and that forms broad national and transnational alliances to fight for social acceptance and public recognition.
>
> (Bauer, 2014: 20)

It is worth noting that all of the participants were more of the new than the old guard, although none of them referred to it as such – the old guard is largely considered anachronistic and outdated, even if some of the aesthetics are still appreciated.

The aforementioned stigma is in part due to the discourse that BDSM and being 'kinky' is pathological, a mental illness. While this discourse remains largely dominant in lots of way, changes to the DSM-IV state that engagement with BDSM is not in itself pathological unless it causes distress to oneself (American Psychiatric Association, 2013).[12] Much of this shift has come from sustained work – whether research, activism, or both – from within kink communities. However it is worth noting perhaps, that in moving away from pathologizing kink, the focus on power relations has led to pain within BDSM being quietly shuffled off to one side even within writing which takes a depathologizing turn – in Kleinplatz and Moser's edited volume *Sadomasochism: Powerful Pleasures* (2006), pain is not listed in the index at all, while in Taylor and Ussher's (2001) discourse analysis of SM, pain is mentioned across discursive themes, but it is not in itself a theme they identify when participants talk about their SM practices. In *Safe, Sane and Consensual* (Langdridge and Barker, 2007), pain is discussed in only one chapter, as 'the unspeakable' (Langdridge, 2007). Pain is not necessarily a central feature of all BDSM – indeed there are plenty of activities that involve no pain at all (Langdridge, 2007; Weinberg, 2006) – but nonetheless erotic pain remains firmly associated with BDSM in the normative discourse, with a great deal of discomfort all around.[13]

Much of the work moving away from pathological perspectives is spread across various disciplines, and it should be noted that kink communities have a "complex and contradictory nature… in which some elements seek to merely extend 'everyday' sexuality whilst others seek to provide an alternative that challenges and confronts" (Langdridge and Butt, 2004: 45), some communities present kink practices as forms of legitimized violence as well as acts of love and playful eroticism, as well as the aforementioned split along identity/practice lines. These presentations can be seen as paralleled to the responsible homosexual versus dangerous queer discourse (Smith, 1992), with the good kinkster versus the bad edge-player and bad queer sharing a complex and convoluted bed.[14]

In this good/bad dichotomy, the good kinkster is one whose practices could be described as 'extending' sexuality; their practices are erotic, and performed within consensual committed relationships which otherwise fit within the bounds of hetero- or homo-normative; their practices carry no risk of long-term bodily damage when done 'safely.' Within this, we can include those who might well not view their practices as kinky at all – more 'spicing things up' – and even those who might be horrified to discover that their practices are regarded as kinky at all. In contrast, the bad edge-player is one whose kinks involve bloodletting, urine and/or feces, sharp edges, breath play, and non-erotic, uncommitted or otherwise non-normative relationships,[15] and those whose practices run the risk of scarring, or otherwise seriously injuring – or even killing – those taking the submissive/slave role. The latter practices are certainly regarded as dangerous even within kink communities – and the acceptability varies hugely. There is, of course, room to acknowledge and unpick how this is not a strict binary, and how breath play has become more normalized in non-kinky sex – but also that the moral panic around choking (which is one form of breath play) and 'rough sex' has undoubtedly fed from the construction of kink as perverted, and longstanding anti-porn feminist discourses. This is not the place to do that, however – we would be here forever.

Langdridge and Butt (2004) posit that acceptance of BDSM in some media versus non-acceptance in governmental policy is possibly due to the emphasis on the sexual in many media portrayals, rather than love and responsibility; these media portrayals can also be read as a fetishization of BDSM itself, a voyeuristic and commercializing approach that does little to benefit BDSM practitioners or those seeking knowledge over titillation (Barker, 2013). Beckman observes that:

> Decontextualized elements of SM and of fetish culture have become integrated for profit. However, while this development on the one hand opens up possibilities of engagement and transgression of the realm of normatively imposed ideas about what constitutes normal sexuality, it is crucial to reflect on capitalism's tendency to facilitate the commodification of apparently 'kinky' sex.
>
> (Beckmann, 2014: 109)

Commodified elements of BDSM – often overlapping with those Newmahr refers to as 'pornonormative' (2011) – tend to be reserved for conventionally attractive, young, hetero- and homo-normative couples, broadly fitting the good kinkster discourse, and instead of including kink in normative sexuality, further reinforces the binary between normative-good and abnormal-bad sexualities and sexual practices.

Within kink communities and activities, there are a series of normative constructions around who does kink, in terms of who can or should play in shared or (semi)public spaces. Some of these constructions may be pornonormative in terms of what aspects of play are marked as 'erotic' or 'sexy'[16] (Newmahr, 2011). Pornonormative constructions of kink are largely focused on visual aspects, on achieving a certain visual aesthetic in terms of how bodies look, having the 'right' clothes and equipment, but are also about what acts constitute kink play. Pornonormative play is intended as erotic – there is no space for kink that is not about eroticism – fitting into normative constructions of the masculine-dominant and the feminine-submissive, with play that is intended to titillate an audience and the players, rather than explore or challenge the power in a relationship. Other normative constructions may depend instead on the domination of clubs and public play spaces by white, non-disabled, middle class people (Bauer, 2007, 2014; Beckmann, 2005; Cruz, 2016; Langdridge and Barker, 2007; Santilla et al., 2002); these aspects often tie into pornonormative constructions of kink – particularly when it comes to acquiring particular equipment, or being able to play publicly without one's presence or actions being called into question.

The discursive construction of kink as play (albeit play that needs to be worked at as serious leisure (Weiss, 2011)) can be read as further removing pain from a position of importance in practices, as there is a jarring disconnect of wider constructions whereby pain is situated against play and enjoyment. Play "references recreation and leisure, and evokes a romantic sense of innocence and freedom from encumbrances" (Newmahr, 2011: 8); this can be tied to a sense of fantasy that is often observed to be a mainstay of kink play and kink scenes (Cruz, 2016; Langdridge and Barker, 2007; Newmahr, 2011; Weiss, 2011), while pain references the unavoidability of everyday life, and the violence of unequal power relations that exist outside of carefully staged unequal power relations in kink. Put simply, pain and play don't mix well in the discourse.

The scripting of kink play scenes[17] relies on social context and social power relations that give specific contextual meanings to play scenes (Weinberg, 2006), so while these scenes may be about the rejection of dominant norms, they are also socially controlled and formed by them (Plante, 2006; Weiss, 2011). Scenes use dominant norms (such as how dominance or violence is performed, with what instruments, or in what setting) as well as playing with them, testing their limits, or challenging their performativity – for example, medical play challenges the norms of the medical setting (when everyday medicine is firmly desexualized) but also relies on the demarcation of certain instruments, clothes, or language as 'medical' in order to indicate what norms are being challenges, as well as appeal to the participants' desires and pleasures.

Kink and Disability

Within various kink scenes of different types, preferences, and locations, disabled people are active participants but not necessarily 'typical' scene members; some scenes situate disabled people primarily as receivers of charity by their fundraisers (Beckmann, 2005) – in the UK, notably through the Sex Maniacs' Ball and Outsiders Club. Some scenes and scene members may be explicitly welcoming to or inclusive of disabled people,[18] but others may be less so – especially scenes which emphasize pornonormative displays of sexuality, where desirable partners tend to be non-disabled and normatively attractive. Of my participants, some did join their local scene and found it welcoming, while others found it less so, particularly when events were not held in wheelchair-accessible spaces, or when their nearest events involved traveling longer distances.

Within some kink scenes, as in wider society, there is often the perception that disabled people only have romantic and sexual relationships with other disabled people (Gillespie-Sells et al., 1998; Shakespeare et al., 1996), or that those who have relationships with disabled people are devotees, or disability fetishists – although there is broader acceptance of disability fetishes within kink. The participants had a mix of romantic and play relationships, with disabled and non-disabled partners. Edward's play partner at the time of the first interview was also disabled, which affected the practicalities of their play together, but that he saw as largely unimportant in terms what he desired in a partner, while Natalie and Rita found that having a disabled partner helped communication within their relationships – which combined romantic intimacy with kink play. It is interesting to note that both women had previously been in abusive relationships with non-disabled men, in which they were forced to engage in BDSM; both placed high importance on being able to effectively communicate in order to practice kink once again. For Natalie, having a shared experience of embodied as well as broader social disablement (she and her husband have the same diagnostic label), and hence of being abject and regarded as abnormal, made her feel more able to trust her partner, but also able to engage in power play. Natalie feels that the shared experience of bodily limitations and capability has meant that they have a greater awareness of how strong they both feel when sexually aroused, but also that she is able to trust him enough to be submissive, as he has also experienced what it is to be powerless as a disabled person.

Bodyminds in kink and bodies in disability are unruly, uncivilized bodyminds (Beckmann, 2005); when disabled bodies engage in kink, they do not become *more* uncivilized (as bodies are either uncivilized or not), but they reimagine what it means to be sexual and what it means to be in pain. Flanagan and Rose's BDSM art performances are examples of this;

> Flanagan and Rose produce meaning that sustains Flanagan's life with and in the disabled body and opens the possibilities to enjoy this body and to derive pleasure from it for both himself and his partner. Cultivating the (eroticized) pain in the S/M practices (both public and private), becomes not a

> matter of simple domination or control of the pain, but a much more complex strategy of transforming and integrating the pain … [and] turning it into a subject-matter of his "technologies of the self" (Foucault, 1988).
>
> (Kolářová, 2010: 49)

For the participants, integrating pain through kink – and integrating kink through pain – was often less publicly performed than Flanagan's artistic work, but was nonetheless a part of their reimagining of their selves as people living with chronic pain. Bauer (2014) argues that kink, as a "sexuality of excess" purposefully denies and resists explanation – rejects 'why'? (as does Flanagan in his poem *Why* (2000)) – with pleasure serving in and for itself alone, but also feels that certain forms of BDSM play maintain the status quo and reinforces (rather than challenges) established power differentials; "a simple philosophy of hedonism without social and environmental responsibilities as integral components would do more harm than good in the 21st century" (Bauer, 2014: 248). Instead, Bauer's participants tried

> To create pleasurable yet responsible ways of confusing boundaries in order to open up bodies and connect across differences. While this may seem less exciting to some theorists, I hold that ethical and political considerations, most basically understood as taking into account and being accountable for the consequences of one's actions, such as the effects on others, social contexts and 'natural' environments, are indispensable.
>
> (Bauer, 2014: 248)

This is echoed in my own participants' narratives – it is not just about pleasure, but also about situating the self in multiple contexts.

Julie, whose relationship with her pain and with kink was fraught – and unhappy due to her limitations – wanted to find ways to be fragile while also engaging in play, although she foresaw it as requiring flexibility and thought on both her part and on her partners' part;

> *Both me and others have to be careful. I don't think they realize how careful at times, but those who I am involved with regularly manage to understand my limitations day-by-day. I think it is fairly obvious in my vocabulary and voice as to how fragile I'm feeling that day.*
>
> (Julie, interview 2)

This using and contesting of her fragility and limitations by Julie is a part of her reconstitution of the self, of controlling her body again – but also about living with pain, making the pain a part of her, even though it makes her body unreliable, and has had a huge impact on her life. Pain and disability push Julie to become a misfit, a mismatch between "the co-constituting relationship between flesh and environment" (Garland-Thomson, 2011: 594), but it also gives her the time and space to become, if not comfortable, then accepting.

Another example of this accepting, and of making pain one of the technologies of the self, is in Natalie and her partner's life, where they have made use of the concept of safe words – words or actions used during BDSM play to communicate needs without breaking the scene, or to put a quick stop to the scene. Safe words are not unproblematic – there can be pressure to not use them, or to make a boast of not having them (Newmahr, 2011) – but they can serve fairly effectively as a way of communicating needs, as Natalie explained;

> [husband] *and I have long used safe-words during non-sexual physical contact. So, an obvious one is tickling or similar messing about, but also if we're any hugging or stroking or just lying entangled with one another, we have words when things become suddenly too painful (i.e., when there's no time or capacity to say, 'Do you mind stopping that now? It's hurting.'). We rarely use safe words in sex – they're there, and they're there for all kinds of sex (since any position or activity risks becoming suddenly very uncomfortable). However, I thought this might be a useful example of something where chronic pain and kink interact; we have thought about safe-words because of kink, but we got good at using them through living with chronic pain (I would say fluent but I can't claim we're perfect with this – we still sometimes say 'Do you mind…' when we're feeling, 'Aaagh, get off!).*
>
> (Natalie, interview 2)

The queering/cripping of pain – of making pain work for and with oneself – is a queering/cripping of the performance of being abjected, it is embracing abjection, embracing a queer and crip selfhood. This same performance can be seen in Flanagan's work, which:

> Embraces the abjected disability. And while the sexual practices of S/M enable Flanagan to transform his physical pain, his engagement with queerness exceeds his individual body (in pain) and stretches to the level of the socially inflected pain of stigma. The transgressive potential of Flanagan's queer gesture thus lies precisely in embracing the disability and sickness to become Sick/Crip.
>
> (Kolářová, 2010: 45)

For the participants, embracing abjection does not mean performing abjection for the non-disabled, but accepting that they are already, and always, abject under the ableist gaze – and thus they can embrace disability and make it work for them, accept its limitations and discomforts and leaks as a part of their self.

Some of the participants also felt that being disabled helped them embrace kink – and vice versa. Edward's comfort with his kink identity was clear in his interviews, and while some of that may be due to the length of time he has been involved in kink, having been playing since his twenties and now in his late forties, it is also due to his disability meaning he does not have to perform normative masculinity. In effect, Edward's disability means he is already disqualified for masculinity, and thus he feels more able to engage in activities that are not properly masculine – such as being a submissive slave to his mistress. This is not to say Edward does not perform masculinity in other ways – such as in his job, or his clothing – but that he is already situated in a place of failure to be a 'proper man' – so why not enjoy it. Natalie's experience was similar, she felt that being bisexual (and particularly being aware that she fancied girls as a young teenager) meant that she had had the option of normality 'taken away' – and thus she was able to embrace disability; embracing disability and bisexuality then meant she was able to embrace kink. Natalie has made being queer/crip work *for* her, and by embracing her multiple failures of normativity, she has opened up a space for her acceptance of her self.

Charlie felt that there were multiple factors affecting their ability to accept and embrace their disability;

> *And I think... so, an existing disability helped me cope with a disability, which is just another layer again, in that sense. Yeah. So, you know, the things that can help people cope can be disability as well. And, yeah, coping with... I mean, there's interactions between everything. I think I was able to resist the medicalization of non-conforming gender because of my experience as a disabled person and trying to navigate and resist some of the medicalization, my awareness of the social model of disability, and just, you know, what kind of medicalized sort of perspectives were going to get applied to my body because I'm non-gender-conforming. I had to resist those. So different things... Yeah.*
>
> (Charlie, interview 2)

This is not to say that all disabled people desire to embrace non-normative sexualities; instead, there is often a drive to emphasize their normative sexuality – especially in what Natalie described as '*disabled people have sex too!*' articles and programs – by making a pronounced performance of their straightness (or homo-normativity), or continually expressing their desire to 'live normal lives.' This almost-exaggerated performance reassures non-disabled people that disabled people are not *totally* monstrous (although it also serves to reinforce their difference – they would not need to reaffirm their normality if they were normal in the first place) and that normality is desirable, and also serves to reinforce to other disabled people that performing normality, and desire of normality, is the best – indeed only – way to live with disability.

Kink and Pain

Pain, like other challenging and confronting practices in kink, is a part of the unspeakable, dangerous, bad side of kink, one that is difficult to portray as 'normal' particularly once it moves away from lighter pain play that runs little to no risk of bodily harm (and might instead be termed sensation play – practices such as light spanking and pinching) toward the heavier, and therefore risker, practices, which carry risks of bruising, breaking the skin, or scarring. The good kinkster plays with sensation, while the bad edge-player uses pain and violence. While this essentializes pain in kink, the unspeakable part of pain means that aspects of kink practices that engage with pain, and confront and challenge constructs of pain are largely silenced – and certainly not discussed with outsiders. This practice of silencing means that kink pain is divorced from other pain through discourses within the subculture. But because pain is still perceived to be a negative experience (due to both kink-specific discourses discussed earlier, and the wider discourses discussed in Chapters 1 and 2), it is pain and its association with violence that allows for kink to be pathologized.

Considering painful play – and play that causes pain – may be too close to pathologizing for comfort, particularly when attempting to present a 'good kinkster' representation of kink practices. Within the various scenes and communities, the opposition of pain and violence against eroticism and play makes a "conscious and deliberate relationship between the erotic and the violent… ethically unacceptable" (Newmahr, 2011: 126), even within sadomasochism. As Newmahr observes, this leads to a difficult and problematic relationship whereby pain is often reconceptualized as not 'really' violence or pain, but instead as a performance of violence, a simulation, complete with symbolic trappings that situate violence and pain within otherwise non-sexual contexts, some requiring a degree of 'make-believe' role-play. This is perhaps in part of the problem of pain, and how kink problematizes the relationship between pain and violence; when pain is considered to be the result of violence, and that as violence is positioned as negative, as uncivilized, then pain must also be negative and uncivilized – a pairing that practitioners must retreat from in order to avoid kink practices as being perceived of as negative and uncivilized (any more than they already are). This conscious stepping away from pain and violence as a central part of many, if not all, kink practices places practitioners in a complex position, where they must legitimize their desire to experience and/or cause pain, while also distancing themselves from the self-same narratives and norms which describe the imbalances of power that characterize the social contexts they challenge and play with; they can only be *playing* if they have first proclaimed that 'this is not us' – once they have disavowed their own place within social power relations. This disavowal-before-play is similar to the relationship kink has with traditional/mainstream models of masculinity; before playing with masculinity, practitioners first recognize the problems of the performance – and thus their masculinity during play is in the way of a parody, and a disavowal, just as the pain in play is also a disavowal of the violence and unequal power relations in traditional/mainstream heterosexuality. We see this as well through the disdain with which – particularly in queer or pansexual kink communities – those men who do ascribe to hegemonic norms of masculinity outside of play are held, particularly when those men[19] however unwittingly behave in ways akin to the *One True Dom* archetype.

Newmahr (2011), in her ethnographic study of a BDSM community in San Francisco, identified multiple reframings and discursive twists through which participants legitimize experiencing and causing pain. The first of these, the *transformed pain* discourse;

> Relies on a conceptualization of pain as an objective stimulus which may or may not result in the feelings of hurt… This 'processing' of pain sensations as pleasurable, within seconds or less, fuels a discourse in which pain can be real but not bad…[Reconciling] masochism with rational thought; if pain does not 'really hurt,' it is depathologised, and therefore it's enjoyment is unproblematic.
>
> (ibid., 2011: 135)

Transformed pain is regarded as not *really* pain, and it is the performative nature of BDSM which allows it to be thus, in the same way that the dominant participant is only dominant with the consent of the submissive, the bound participant is easily freed, and the age-player's nappy is not needed once the scene ends. This depathologizing relies on the recognition of performance and play, but also on the explicit denial of the construction of pain in the scene (or of dominance, of bodily restriction, or of incontinence). In order for pain to be transformed, the person experiencing pain must first recognize themselves as not normally in pain and that pain is normally bad and unwanted. It also relies on a conception of pain akin to the Specificity Theory,[20] where pain is straightforward somatic sensation – and it is only the conscious interpretation of that sensation which marks it as pain. This reframing is also commonly found in the 'good kinkster' reframing of kink, as one which uses sensation for erotic gratification, but denies that the sensation may be produced through violence.

Aspects of Newmahr's transformed pain could be identified in parts of how my participants spoke about kink, sex, and pain – such as when Natalie described kink and sex as:

> *The opposite to illness – the latter makes my body feel ugly, useless and thoroughly dysfunctional but sex (these days) makes me feel beautiful, physically stronger and useful both to myself and* [my partner].
>
> (Natalie, interview 1)

As a space to engage positively with her body, in a way that works *with*, rather than against, its limitations and capabilities, sex and kink gives Natalie a great deal of self-confidence. In this way we can understand her seeing kink pain as transformative – not such in terms of pain as 'not really pain' but in terms of pain as being transformed from a negative experience into something else. This was a theme that ran through several participants' interviews, whereby kink practices help to construct a space in which the limitations and capabilities of the body can be explored;

> *The focusing pain calms me, the sensations aren't as deep and pervasive as in chronic pain, the pain is specific. I can appreciate it changing sensations, the*

> *pain peaking and troughing. I react in many ways to kink pain, it invigorates me, it turns me on, it allows me to breathe deep full happy breaths. My body doesn't cope very well to non-kink, non-chronic pain, it tends to exaggerate the sensations, making a papercut seem highly painful. It goes into shut down mode quite quickly in these situations.*
>
> (Julie, interview 2)

Newmahr's second reframing of pain, termed *sacrificial pain*, was found particularly in discipline and punishment scenes, and situates pain as a sacrifice on the part of the bottom for the good of and desires of the top; it is the top, the dominant, who is the sadist, or who needs to express a part of themselves through activities which cause pain for others; the submissive endures but does not enjoy, with their endurance acting as a form of service to their dominant. Newmahr (2011) observed this as a particularly gendered discourse, frequently expressed by submissive women in D/s relationships; it is less easy to align this reframing with the 'good kinkster' – particularly when the otherwise 'good' kinkster is one who challenges normative constructions of gender and power imbalances – but it is echoed in discourse which position the dominant practitioner as having a particular knowledge and/or skill-set that enables them to 'know' what the submissive needs, and if the submissive endures to a particular point, they will be themselves transformed, or able to access the place in which pain is no longer anything other than sensation.

Julie, in addition to engaging with transformative framing of pain, enjoys the performance of submission, and draws on a more sacrificial understanding of pain in submission. Her enjoyment of submission means that kink play is pleasurable, even though the experience of pain is not. In this way, her kink play creates a space for re-engaging with the body and somatic sensation in ways that are both pleasurable and painful. The control of pain and bodies practiced by the participants seeks not to control the pain directly (as it would be through pain medication or pain reduction techniques) but instead to control what can be controlled; namely their bodies' responses to pleasure and new, temporary, pain.

> *Kink pain is about proving otherwise. It's about laying yourself vulnerable, and opening yourself up to your own strength and the strength of others. You are giving something away, but similarly getting so much back. And testing your own resolve. Because in any kink pain situation, you can stop it if it gets too much – even if you then regret it moments later. Chronic pain is nothing of the sort. It tests you. It can, however much you rise above it to get through it, bring you crashing down. And you can't say a safe word and step away from it. It makes you fragile, to some extent.*
>
> (Julie, diary entry)

For Julie, the key difference between kink pain and chronic pain – strength versus fragility – is down to control; chronic pain makes her fragile, because she cannot control it (and we'll come to control in subsequent chapters). The experience of disability can often be one of powerlessness, and vulnerability – even if powerlessness and vulnerability are only imposed by others, rather than a condition of bodily capabilities and limitations – and in constructing a space where one's vulnerability can be tested, however artificially, kink play is a space where Julie is *not* vulnerable or fragile, but strong and desirable. Similarly, Natalie explained in her second interview that kinky sex is therapeutic for her on some level – it is a space of recovery, and positive bodily experience. This framing of kink pain as therapeutic was missing from Newmahr's account, and there is deep discomfort within kink communities in framing kink in terms of therapeutic terms (Barker et al., 2007) – in discussing how engaging with kink might be unintentionally therapeutic (in that the person is not practicing kink *as a therapy*, or because they have thought that getting flogged might in some way help their trauma – but it is a happy side effect).

The third reframing discourse Newmahr identified is equally as gendered, with *investment pain* as a hyper masculine discourse which promises future rewards. This is most frequently paralleled within discourses of pain and reward in sports. Investment pain "is understood not merely as an unfortunate by-product, but as a means to a particular end. While hurting is not the goal, in and of itself, it is rewarding for both what it evidences and what it produces" (Newmahr, 2011: 138). This pain is not experienced or endured for the sake of others, and is not sought out by either bottom or top, but is instead a mark of one's ability to achieve a particular state. This is echoed in the knowing dominant/naive submissive construction discussed above, particularly in terms of pain being transformative and itself transformed, but the process of enduring is in itself important – the process of being able to take it better, to last longer, to be better.

This framing in terms of exploring one's limits was present in other participants' narratives. For Rita, Charlie and David, the control over their pain is framed around their wish for a sense of endurance, and of having pushed their limits. Rita explained;

> *I mean, one of the things I get most out of play, of kink play of all kinds, when I'm subbing is a feeling of achievement. Kind of a feeling I've done things well, which both my partners are very good about reinforcing at every opportunity. And especially when I spend quite a lot of my time being bed-ridden and a lot of my time being … inconvenienced by pain and fatigue that… you know, to be able to go, well, I took that… you know, I took that caning, and it was actually hell, but I feel so good about having been able to do it. It is a really, really powerful thing.*
>
> (Rita, interview 1)

For Charlie and David, the sense of achievement which they both feel on having incurred consensual pain is one in which they are reminded of their bodily ability and strength, of a sense of mind over matter, which is denied to them through living with chronic pain.

Newmahr identified only one discourse, very much in the minority, whereby pain and the relationship with it is framed in positive terms; in what she has termed *autotelic pain* (2011), pain is liked *as pain*, for pain's sake. For those who situated pain as autotelic:

> The pain hurts, but hurt also feels good. Participants who frame pain in this way have an extraordinarily difficult time articulating their experience of pain. They generally distinguish between kinds of pain that they do like and kinds of pain that they do not like; the particular kind of pain, rather than the context, determines whether the response is favorable … Among these participants, eroticism is often denied or recast. Most of the people who say that they like to hurt or be hurt also say that SM is not sexual for them. And those who do use the word 'hurt' draw the line between 'hurt' and 'harm' with the distinction being largely temporal; harm is lasting.
>
> (ibid., 2011: 139–140)

This discourse relies on, and reinforces, the positioning of pain and violence as the antithesis of pleasure and eroticism; rather than denying the painful aspect of kink practices, practitioners instead deny the erotic – and continue this previously-discussed framing of kink whereby violence and eroticism cannot exist together. This discourse of autotelic pain is perhaps closest to what we would recognize as 'true' masochism, the enjoyment of pain and denigration for its own sake, in that it conceives of pain as painful. However, as it has nonetheless been shown that state of mind and intent alters the experience of painful events (Kleinplatz and Moser, 2006), it is just as conceivable that people who reframe kink pain as not painful are not experiencing the pain we understand as the result of injury or violence. Despite Newmahr's (2011) work, pain as an embodied experience, as a bodily experience for kink practitioners, remains largely side-lined by considerations of power and of the legal standing of kink. While I posit that this is due to a degree of discomfort with problematic relationship between pain, violence and play, it is also undoubtedly due to the relatively small size of the field when it comes to academic enquiry into BDSM.

Notes

1 Or sometimes *kink(y) play*.

2 There is lots of space here for BDSM to be considered outside of/beyond sexuality, but that is a discussion somewhat beyond the discourse where BDSM is associated with sexual behavior.

3 This is not to say that there are no asexual people – but instead that asexuality is imposed against their will and desires as sexual people.

4 While heteronormative sex has arguably become more kinky, the limits are still relatively narrow, and rarely stray beyond what Newmahr refers to as the 'pornonormative' (2011).

5 We see the self-same argument used against LGBTQ+ inclusive sex and relationship education in schools: it will encourage children to have non-heteronormative sex.

6 This can perhaps best be defined as: 'I find that person sexy *because* of their disability' or 'I find that disability sexy' rather than 'I find that person sexy.'

7 Deservedly. Some devotees tend to objectify disabled people, rather than viewing them as *people*.
8 This does, however, contrast with the discussion around disabled cishet men's 'right' to sexual activity and the employment of sex workers; see Liddiard (2019).
9 There are issues here – see the next paragraph.
10 Smooth transition here, hope you enjoyed that.
11 The art of Tom of Finland being an excellent example of this aesthetic.
12 Engaging in BDSM, kink, and/or fetish practices was defined as a psychiatric condition by the DSM until 2013 (Gerson, 2015; Wright, 2018); the combination of pathologization and criminalization of consensual kink is much more longstanding (Beckmann, 2009, 2014; Langdridge and Barker, 2007).
13 Literally, sometimes.
14 For an idea of how convoluted, observe the 'does kink belong at pride' online discourse. Do so at your own risk.
15 From play-only relationships, paid sex work and pro Dom/me services to scenarios such as 24/7 D/s play.
16 Slim, large-breasted women in PVC catsuits, lingerie, waxed or shaven genitalia, and so on and so forth – the imagery often associated with pornographic depictions of BDSM.
17 'Scenes' here refers to the scenario and space of a particular interaction, rather than the other use of 'scene' in kink, which refers to the communities and spaces/places – the subculture. This is absolutely not confusing *at all*.
18 For example, discussing wheelchair and other physical access, or including visibly disabled people in images.
19 Somewhere a faint cry of 'not all men!' is heard, and roundly ignored.
20 See Chapter 1.

References

Aguilera RJ (2000) Disability and Delight: Staring Back at the Devotee Community. *Sexuality and Disability* 18(4): 255–261.

American Psychiatric Association (2013) *Diagnostic and Statistical Manual of Mental Disorders: DSM-V.* 5th ed. Washington, DC: American Psychiatric Association.

Bahner J (2021) *Sexual Citizenship and Disability: Understanding Sexual Support in Policy, Practice and Theory.* London: Routledge.

Baldwin G (1991) 'Old Guard': Its Origins, Traditions, Mystique & Rules. *Drummer Magazine.* Available at: http://www.evilmonk.org/a/oldguard.cfm.

Barker M (2013) Consent Is a Grey Area? A Comparison of Understandings of Consent in Fifty Shades of Grey and on the BDSM blogosphere. *Sexualities* 16(8): 896–914.

Barker M, Gupta C and Iantaffi A (2007) The Power of Play: The Potentials and Pitfalls in Healing Narratives of BDSM. In: Barker M and Langdridge D (eds) *Safe, Sane & Consensual: Contemporary Perspectives of Sadomasochism.* Basingstoke: Palgrave Macmillan, pp. 197–216.

Bauer R (2007) Playgrounds & New Territories: The Potential of BDSM Practices to Queer Genders. In: Barker M and Langdridge D (eds) *Safe, Sane & Consensual: Contemporary Perspectives of Sadomasochism.* Basingstoke: Palgrave Macmillan, pp. 177–194.

Bauer R (2014) *Queer BDSM Intimacies: Critical Consent and Pushing Boundaries.* Basingstoke: Palgrave Macmillan.

Beckmann A (2005) Representing 'Healthy' and 'Sexual' Bodies: the Media, 'Disability' and Consensual 'SM'. In: King M and Watson K (eds) *Representing Health: Discourses of Health and Illness in the Media.* Basingstoke: Palgrave Macmillan, pp. 206–233.

Beckmann A (2009) *The Social Construction of Sexuality and Perversion: Deconstructing Sadomasochism.* Basingstoke: Palgrave Macmillan.

Beckmann A (2014) Sadomasochism. In: Atkinson R (ed) *Shades of Deviance: A Primer on Crime, Deviance and Social Harm.* Abingdon: Routledge, pp. 108–111.

Boehmer U (2002) Twenty Years of Public Health Research: Inclusion of Lesbian, Gay, Bisexual, and Transgender Populations. *American Journal of Public Health* 92(7): 1125–1130. DOI: 10.2105/AJPH.92.7.1125.

Branstrom R and van der Star A (2013) All inclusive Public Health—What about LGBT Populations? *The European Journal of Public Health* 23(3): 353–354. DOI: 10.1093/eurpub/ckt054.

Coulter RWS, Kenst KS, Bowen DJ, et al. (2014) Research Funded by the National Institutes of Health on the Health of Lesbian, Gay, Bisexual, and Transgender Populations. *American Journal of Public Health* 104(2): e105–e112. DOI: 10.2105/AJPH.2013.301501.

Crossan R and Monaghan K (2013) Ouch Talk Show 100: Sex and Relationships Special (10th September 2013). *Ouch! Disability Talk Show 100.* Available at: http://www.bbc.co.uk/podcasts/series/ouch (accessed 12 September 2013).

Cruz A (2016) *The Color of Kink: Black Women, BDSM, and Pornography.* New York: NYU Press.

Flanagan B, Juno A and Vale V (2000) *Bob Flanagan: Supermasochist.* RE/Search People Series. New York: Juno Books.

Foucault M (1988) Truth, Power, Self. An Interview with Michel Foucault. In: Martin LH, Gutman H and Hutton PH (eds) *Technologies of the Self: A Seminar with Michel Foucault.* London: Tavistock Press, pp. 9–15.

Garland-Thomson R (2011) Misfits: A Feminist Materialist Disability Concept. *Hypatia* 26(3): 591–609. DOI: 10.1111/j.1527-2001.2011.01206.x.

Gerson MN (2015) BDSM Versus the DSM. *The Atlantic*, 13 January. Available at: https://www.theatlantic.com/health/archive/2015/01/bdsm-versus-the-dsm/384138/.

Gillespie-Sells K, Hill M and Robbins B (1998) *She Dances to Different Drums: Research into Disabled Women's Sexuality.* London: King's Fund.

Goodley D, Lawthom R, Liddiard K, et al. (2019) Provocations for Critical Disability Studies. *Disability & Society* 34(6): 972–997. DOI: 10.1080/09687599.2019.1566889.

Greenwall A and Hough S (2008) Culture and Disability in Sexuality Studies: A Methodological and Content Review of Literature. *Sexuality and Disability* 26: 189–196.

Guldin A (2000) Self-Claiming Sexuality: Mobility Impaired People & American Culture. *Sexuality and Disability* 18(4): 233–238.

Kafer A (2013) *Feminist, Queer, Crip.* Bloomington and Indianapolis: Indiana University Press.

Kleinplatz PJ and Moser C (eds) (2006) *Sadomasochism: Powerful Pleasures.* Binghampton, NY: Harrington Park Press.

Kolářová K (2010) Performing the Pain: Opening the (Crip) Body for (Queer) Pleasures. *Review of Disability Studies* 6(3): 44–52.

Kumari Campbell F (2009) *Contours of Ableism: The Production of Disability and Abledness.* Basingstoke: Palgrave Macmillan.

Langdridge D (2007) Speaking the Unspeakable: S/M & the Eroticisation of Pain. In: Barker M and Langdridge D (eds) *Safe, Sane & Consensual: Contemporary Perspectives of Sadomasochism.* Basingstoke: Palgrave Macmillan, pp. 85–97.

Langdridge D and Barker M (2007) Situating Sadomasochism. In: Barker M and Langdridge D (eds) *Safe, Sane & Consensual: Contemporary Perspectives of Sadomasochism.* Basingstoke: Palgrave Macmillan, pp. 3–9.

Langdridge D and Butt T (2004) A Hermeneutic Phenomenological Investigation of the Construction of Sadomasochistic Identities. *Sexualities* 7(1): 31–53. DOI: 10.1177/1363460704040137.

Liddiard K (2019) *The Intimate Lives of Disabled People*. Abingdon: Routledge.

Mailhot Amborski A, Bussières E-L, Vaillancourt-Morel M-P, et al. (2022) Sexual Violence Against Persons With Disabilities: A Meta-Analysis. *Trauma, Violence, & Abuse* 23(4): 1330–1343. DOI: 10.1177/1524838021995975.

McRuer R and Mollow A (2012) Introduction. In: McRuer R and Mollow A (eds) *Sex and Disability*. Durham, NC: Duke University Press, pp. 1–34.

Newmahr S (2011) *Playing on the Edge: Sadomasochism, Risk, and Intimacy*. Bloomington: Indiana University Press.

Office for National Statistics (2019) *Disability and crime, UK: 2019*. Available at: https://www.ons.gov.uk/peoplepopulationandcommunity/healthandsocialcare/disability/bulletins/disabilityandcrimeuk/2019 (accessed 1 February 2023).

Plante RF (2006) Sexual Spanking, the Self, and the Construction of Deviance. *Journal of Homosexuality* 50(2–3): 59–79.

Rembis MA (2010) Beyond the Binary: Rethinking the Social Model of Disabled Sexuality. *Sexuality and Disability* 28: 51–60.

Rogers C (2009) (S)excerpts from a Life Told: Sex, Gender and Learning Disability. *Sexualities* 12(3): 270–288.

Rubin G (1998) Old Guard, New Guard. *Cuir Underground*. Available at: http://www.black-rose.com/cuiru/archive/4-2/oldguard.html.

Santilla P, Sandnabber NK, Alison L, et al. (2002) Investigating the Underlying Structure in Sadomasochistically Oriented Behavior. *Archives of Sexual Behaviour* 31(2): 185–196.

Shakespeare T, Gillespie-Sells K and Davies D (1996) *The Sexual Politics of Disability: Untold Desires*. London and New York: Cassell.

Shildrick M (2009) *Dangerous Discourses of Disability, Subjectivity and Sexuality*. Basingstoke: Palgrave Macmillan.

Siebers T (2012) A Sexual Culture for Disabled People. In: McRuer R and Mollow A (eds) *Sex and Disability*. Durham, NC: Duke University Press, pp. 37–53.

Smith AM (1992) Resisting the Erasure of Lesbian Sexuality: A Challenge for Queer Activism. In: Plummer K (ed) *Modern Homosexualities: Fragments of Lesbian and Gay Experiences*. London: Routledge, pp. 200–216.

Solvang P (2007) The Amputee Body Desired: Beauty Destabilized? Disability Re-valued? *Sexuality and Disability* 25: 51–64.

Taylor GW and Ussher JM (2001) Making Sense of S&M: A Discourse Analytic Account. *Sexualities* 4(3): 293–314. DOI: 10.1177/136346001004003002.

Tepper MS (2000) Sexuality and Disability: The Missing Discourse of Pleasure. *Sexuality and Disability* 18(4): 283–290.

Treating Autism, ESPA Research and Autism Treatment Plus (2014) *Medical Comorbidities in Autism Spectrum Disorders: A Primer for Health Care Professionals and Policy Makers*. 2nd ed. London: Treating Autism Publications.

Tremain S (2000) Queering Disabled Sexuality Studies. *Sexuality and Disability* 18(4): 291–299.

Verschuren JEA, Enzlin P, Dijkstra PU, et al. (2010) Chronic Disease and Sexuality: A Generic Conceptual Framework. *Journal of Sex Research* 47(2–3): 153–170.

Waxman Fiduccia B (2000) Current Issues in Sexuality and the Disability Movement. *Sexuality and Disability* 18(3): 167–174.

Weinberg TS (2006) Sadomasochism and the Social Sciences: A Review of the Sociological and Social Psychological Literature. *Journal of Homosexuality* 50(2–3): 17–40.

Weiss M (2011) *Techniques of Pleasure: BDSM and the Circuits of Sexuality*. Durham, NC and London: Duke University Press.

Wright S (2018) De-pathologization of Consensual BDSM. *The Journal of Sexual Medicine* 15(5): 622–624. DOI: 10.1016/j.jsxm.2018.02.018.

Zitzelsberger H (2005) (In)visibility: Accounts of Embodiment of Women with Physical Disabilities and Differences. *Disability & Society* 20(4): 389–403. DOI: 10.1080/09687590500086492.

4 Crip Time

Pace of Life

Pace of life is here defined as the speed at which everyday reproductive tasks and normative, capitalist-productive work are required to be performed, as well as the time of day (or night) those tasks or work are expected to be done (Kafer, 2013; Kumari Campbell, 2009; Wendell, 1996). As Wendell (1996) observes, the increases in pace of life in modern neoliberal society – longer working hours, faster travel, quicker movement of information – is resulting in increasing numbers of people who are regarded as disabled; the space of crip time is increasing as a result as more and more people are falling short of being 'on time.' For Ahmed (2006), in writing of the perception of the failure of objects to adequately enable tasks to be completed, she echoes thinking on disabled people – they are failed objects, in that the body is reduced to an object that fails to enable the tasks of work to be completed; disability is a failure of performance in/on time. The life course of a disabled person is different from an able person, as a result of this failure to perform, and because

> certain objects [and 'choices'] are available to us because of lines that we have already taken: our 'life courses' follow a certain sequence, which is also a matter of following a direction or of 'being directed' in a certain way (birth, childhood, adolescence, marriage, reproduction, death).
>
> (ibid., 2006: 21)

Here Ahmed is following Halberstam (2005), applying the concept of orientation to time – the queer body's path through time is oriented differently to the straight body; the crip bodymind's path through time more closely resembles the queer path in its divergence from the norm.

Thinking through pace of life exposes the compulsory ableness behind constructions as apparently disparate as timekeeping, speed (and method) of movement, and development of various 'skills' in childhood; crip time runs alongside Lochlann Jain's (2013) *prognosis time*, the time of life at which diseases appear, the time of terminal illness, between diagnosis and death; the sick body exists in prognosis time, and "the prognosis epitomizes the haunting character of death …

DOI: 10.4324/9781003006237-5

In one swift motion, the cancer prognosis detonates time, which scatters like so many glass shards" (ibid., 2013: 28). Although none of the participants had been given life-limiting (or terminal) diagnoses, both Edward and Julie lived with progressive conditions, and thus live in prognosis time as well as crip time; they have diagnoses that come complete with timescales, bodily selves forever in anticipation of 'worsening' impairment, together with the anticipation of a future remaking of the self, of re-adjusting to another self.

McRuer (2006), Goodley (2014), and many others, myself included, see disability and ableism as situated firmly in the practices of neoliberalism. Neoliberalism, for Tyler (2013), is a context helping to form particular discourses, a form of governance that creates inequalities with public consent, through policies in support of the 'free market,' and without mainstream political opposition; these inequalities cause ongoing financial and social insecurity for those in employment, along with a fear of becoming the abject – with social abjection as the lot of those without incomes or who rely on welfare support. The deliberate precarization (ibid., 2013: 199) of labor insecurity, and the loss of collective agency brought about by increasingly precarious and insecure work across the majority of sectors, is accompanied by increasing demand for 'flexible' laboring bodies (McRuer, 2006); flexible to fit the changing demands of a precarious labor market, but also flexible in order to get ahead, to adapt in ways that mean they are able to continue working and producing. Those flexible bodies – immediately shaped through discourses of neoliberalism, but nonetheless framed in broader ideas of the normal and the ideal – are very specifically *able* at the same time, specifically

> Heterosexual, able-bodied ... [and able to] work with queer and disabled minority, flexibly contracting and expanding, while queer, disabled minorities flexibly comply. Because all of this happens in a discursive climate of tolerance, which values and profits from 'diversity' ... the heterosexual, able-bodied subject, as well as the postmodern culture that produced him or her, can easily disavow how much the subjective contraction and expansion of able-bodied heterosexuality (and ... neoliberal political and economic logics more generally) are actually compliant on queer, disabled bodies.
>
> (ibid., 2006: 18)

For Kumari Campbell, there is a tautology within neoliberalism – the discursive climate of tolerance specific to neoliberalism promotes inclusion, especially when difference can be cast as profitable or consumable, but the ableist discourse of flexible normativity casts disability as "inherently negative, ontologically intolerable and in the end, a dispensable remnant [of uncivilized times]. This casting results in an ontological foreclosure wherein positive signification of disability becomes unspeakable" (ibid., 2009: 12).

Puar (2009), however, situates neoliberalism as a more *direct* cause of failure itself, in that encounters with sociocultural and neoliberal-capitalist infrastructures may render the body's affective capacity inadequate. The effect of neoliberal policies – such as long-term precarious work causing stress and illness – creates what Puar terms debility, as do the constrictions placed on individuals and collective groups by neoliberal discourses. Shildrick identifies debility as inherently profitable;

> it is in the interests of neo-liberalism to produce and sustain bodies as debilitated and therefore susceptible to a range of market commodities that hold out the promise of therapeutic interventions into the relative failures of physical, cognitive and affective embodiment.
>
> (Shildrick, 2015: 11)

thus disability becomes failure to use those commodities – a failure of self-control – even though access to these may not be equitable and may not be appropriate.

Debility presents both danger and opportunity to think through the notion of pacing, and the impact of pace of life on bodies positioned as both disabled and not. Opportunity, because the notion of debility, as a way of thinking about how the pace of life impacts on bodies and lived experience, arguably "[affords] greater recognition of geo-social forces and circuits" (Wearing et al., 2015: 2), but also a danger, as "concepts such as impairment and debility do not indicate new modes of egalitarianism but, rather, operate as a superficial rebranding of medicalized paradigms" (Inckle, 2015: 45). Taking the approach that both views have a measure of value, pacing can be read as a double-edged sword: it gives space to acknowledge that a normal (and ever-increasing) pace of life is impossible to achieve, and instead further debilitates disabled bodies, wearing them down through continual demands to keep up – but pacing can also be read *as* that same demand, as a requirement to perform. Pacing is a performance of a slowed pace of life, but also a performance of refusal to wholly reject the normal pace of life – instead it is a performance of striving for normal through tightly controlling the body.

Puar's conception of debility can also be seen as a loss of function, of ability – and in many ways can be read as acquired disability, in that it is the requirements of modern life that cause a person's impairment to be diagnosed, or the impact of capitalism upon the bodymind, causing loss of capacity over time, through violence and/or environmental damage, the latter leading to illness or developmental disabilities. For Shildrick (2015) debility is concerned with minor but prolific failures of the body or mind; but she is unsure if this approach is useful for disability, especially given that nobody escapes debility in some way. I remain unconvinced that debility always has space for disability, agreeing with Mitchell and Snyder when they observe that "there is not a level playing field that all bodies occupy, and calling for a universalizing recognition of insufficiency will do little to accomplish meaningful systems change" (Mitchell and Snyder, 2015: 29). Debility, in positing an inherently negative view of itself, leaves no space for positive disabled identities – particularly those disabled people who do not experience their disability as a loss – and instead reinforces the ontological *intolerability* of disability, and rather than "[indicating] new modes of egalitarianism …, operate as a superficial rebranding of medicalized paradigms" (Inckle, 2015: 43). Finding a way for debility and disability to work together requires greater engagement with the ways in which disability itself is constituted as a lifelong state, compared to debility's temporary nature, and with thinking around disability engaging with the ways in which the pace of life can be disabling. This is where crip time comes in.

Crip(ping) Time

The ever-increasing pace of life demanded by neoliberal society and 24/7 capitalism (Crary, 2013), which Puar (2009) identifies as causing debility, for Kafer (2013) and Wendell (1996) is instead *disabling.* 24/7 capitalism demands workers who are capable of working hours independent of their local time zone – working early mornings or late nights, or at times that match the working hours of a stock market halfway across the globe – as well as workers who are able to meet continually-increasing expectations and continually-shortening deadlines. This acceleration of the pace of life, which is frequently debilitating for otherwise non-disabled individuals, can be further disabling for disabled people, as

> when the pace of life in a society increases, there is a tendency for more people to become disabled, not only because of physically damaging consequences of efforts to go faster, but also because fewer people can meet expectations of 'normal' performance; the physical (and mental) limitations of those who cannot meet the new pace of life become conspicuous and disabling … for those who must move or think slowly, and for those whose energy is severely limited, expectations of pace can make work, recreational, community, and social activities inaccessible.
>
> (Wendell, 1996: 37–38)

The expectation for performing hetero-normative, flexible, independent, proper bodiliness, at the right time and in the right amount of time is a key aspect of disability, and a disabled body is one that fails to perform in a timely manner, whether it is failing to reach the right childhood developmental milestones at the right times, failing to sustain productivity, or failing to have 'normal' (read: heterosexual, spontaneous, 'vanilla') sex. Crip time, exploring the construction of time through a crip lens, is a somewhat humorous reference to disabled people's frequent need for 'extra time' that

> Might result from a slower gait, a dependency on attendants (who might themselves be running late), malfunctioning equipment (from wheelchairs to hearing aids), a bus driver who refuses to stop for a disabled passenger, or an ableist encounter with a stranger that throws one off schedule. Operating on crip time, then, might be not only about a slower speed of movement but also about ableist barriers over which one has little to no control; in either case, crip time involves an awareness that disabled people might need more time to accomplish something or to arrive somewhere.
>
> (Kafer, 2013: 26)

At the same time, crip time questions notions of 'normal' time – of when something should be done and how long it should take – and how time is itself a part of how disability is constructed. Thus, I would add to Kafer's explanation of crip time notions of what constitutes 'proper' or 'regular' working hours, the notions of developmental milestones, and the experience of needing longer to respond to a question due to a 'slower' thinking process.

For Foucault (1973), time was a key part of the discourse of disease and medicine, both in the clinical gaze and in the progression of disease and recovery. Crip time then can also include diagnosis, prognosis, and progression of illness or impairment – chronic or acute, acquired or congenital, in remission, relapsed – as well as the very notion of prognosis and treatment itself. Development and chronological age are particularly important in terms of a medical diagnosis of disability/impairment in children (Rogers, 2009); asynchronicity between 'mental age' and chronological age is both a common descriptor of cognitive impairment for children, and a cause of discomfort/horror in those with normative expectations. This horror becomes quickly apparent when issues of gender and sexuality come into play, when 'childlike' minds inhabit 'adult' bodies capable of reproduction, and all the emissions and 'mess' reproductive maturity entails – let alone the sexual desires and 'needs' ascribed to sexually mature bodies; Kafer (2013) explores this more thoroughly in how it relates to Ashley X and growth attenuation treatment for 'severely' disabled children.

Medically-framed understandings of disability are oriented through time in not just in terms of progression and prognosis, but also in regarding the future in curative terms; disability, like queer, is counter to progress and civilizing processes (Kafer, 2013), and considerations of the future are frequently disability-free. For Kafer (2013), taking cues from the work of Edelman (2004), the figure of 'the Child' buttresses ableist hetero-normativity – and the future Child cannot be disabled, just as the disabled Child of today must have a better future through rehabilitation, or no future at all. This bleeds into the fear of disabled people's reproductive potential, either as inadequate parents of non-disabled children, or as inadequate parents of disabled children, forcing unwanted disability into the future through procreation.

At a practical level a diagnosis of chronic pain (or another condition, illness, or impairment that includes chronic pain) takes time – sometimes months, sometimes years – to be confirmed by medical professionals. After diagnosis – and sometimes before – more time is needed to access specialist medics, to find appropriate specialist care or medication. This lengthy process, firmly situated in the medical sphere, continually reinforces pain as medical, even as medicine may have little to say about chronic pain. Throughout this, the phenomenological experience of pain – how it feels, how those living with chronic pain experience it – is assumed to be the same. This is, as I will demonstrate, not the case – and the relationship between time and pain is far more complex.

In dividing pain up into chronic and acute, based squarely on temporal terminology, orientated in time toward a normative construction of prognosis and expected recovery, pain is divided into 'normal' and 'abnormal.' While any pain can be regarded as abnormal – in that having no pain and thus being 'healthy' is the normal ideal, and pain is regarded as unwanted or presumed to be the result of injury – the experience of acute pain is a normal event, something all people are presumed to have had. Chronic pain, on the other hand, is *always* wholly abnormal. While in a strictly medical setting, the focus on time is concentrated on dividing the experience of pain into chronic or acute, and there is an assumption that experience of pain is the same as it was when the pain was first felt, when the pain was diagnostically useful or could be regarded as acute – thus chronic pain is cast as a repetition, saying or doing nothing useful or meaningful (Conrad and Muñoz, 2010).

While much theorizing around crip time focuses on the experience of disability in terms of pace of life relating to others, crip time includes a huge range of ways of thinking about time, and ways of performing in/moving through time, that are affected by the composition, comportment, and capacities of the disabled individual's bodymind. When it comes to living with chronic pain, the notion of crip time provides a fertile ground for thinking through the experience of living with chronic pain over months and years, and the relationship between time and pain. Expanding notions of crip time to include experiences of becoming crip – of becoming used to, and accepting of, acquired disability, as well as developing a positive crip identity – can thus explore the tensions between the normal and the crip, rather than viewing crip as wholly separate from – or opposite to – normal. The contestatory nature of crip destabilizes normative notions of time, but also leaves space for ways of being in time – and moving through time – which are less than distinctly crip, which include more normative-seeming ways of being/moving. As being crip can also be understood as *becoming* crip – a process rather than a fixed state, notions of crip time need to have space to include ways of being/moving that are both normative and crip *within the same bodymind* – thus, while some aspects of an individual's ways of being/moving may appear distinctly crip, they may also perform distinctly normative ways of being/moving. In addition, performing normative ways of being in/moving through time may be an important part of an individual's acceptance of their bodymind, a part of their becoming crip, in that they are finding spaces for their bodymind – spaces in which they can feel positively, negatively, neither and both – and perhaps cripping normative ways of being in/moving through time.

Crip time can be expanded to explore the pace of life, its acceleration under neoliberal regimes, and how disabled lives can present as slow and unreliable lives – or a need for a slow life, as ways of doing and thinking slowly (Goodley, 2014; Hickey-Moody, 2015), and as ways of responding to an unreliable bodymind. Conceiving of crip time as a space for unreliability recognizes the possibilities and impossibility of the crip bodymind, while also demonstrating how normative discourses privilege a narrow range of capacities. Acknowledging slow and unreliable lives

> is a way of valuing how 'disabled' bodies and subjectivities experience and reproduce the world. Implicit in this suggestion is the belief that disabled

> [bodyminds] and embodied subjectivities experience and reproduce the world in ways that show up limits in popular sensory and spatial geographies.
>
> (Hickey-Moody, 2015: 140)

Slow and unreliable lives demonstrate how the demands of a normative pace of life are, in many cases, simply normative *demands*, rather than necessities. However, crip time is not always slow – as Price points out, it can also be "accelerated to a terrifying cadence" (2015: 273) in times of crisis. In addition, crip time can include time for diagnosis and prognosis, pace of development of bodily skills (such as walking, continence, or talking) and the normative rejection of a disabled future. Crip time in the context of chronic pain thus includes other aspects of living, particularly the time needed to manage disability, and the reliably unreliable bodymind, to think and do slowly, and to live at a pace that reduces the chance of unwanted or unchosen pain events.

Crip Time as Time to be Unreliable

It is impossible to be in chronic pain and also to maintain a state of constant distress; the reliably unreliable body cannot be forever shut off from the world. Even beyond the need to communicate pain, the participants' narratives all told of a need to continue, to function in the world, to be and to do, while also acknowledging their pain and vulnerabilities. Living with chronic pain changes the lifeworld, but it does not end it. The world may be smaller, the possibilities fewer, the agency further constrained, but life does not end; the phenomenological self continues. Catherine and Julie have found that, over time, their chronic pain has not lessened, but it draws less of their focus; they are able to continue on, to live. As Catherine put it:

> *At the beginning of my illness, I was constantly aware of this same level of pain, but as I sort of got used to it, I stopped being consciously aware... Although there are often signs that I'm unconsciously aware – I'll be moody or snappy or tired. Then some days it's more like, I'm aware of it, but can push it to the background.*
>
> (Catherine, interview 2)

Moodiness and snappiness – and tiredness – are subjective, requiring us to regard ourselves as we would observe another's emotional expression; Catherine is speaking as much of how she expects others to read her emotional expression as she is of her own emotions, ascribing them negative (and gendered) descriptors. Her emotional expression may be due to pain, but it is also due to the difficulty of performing as normal, of performing as pain-free; it is not solely an expression of pain, because she has learnt not to speak of her pain, not to let her pain show – and instead it escapes in the cracks of tone and choice of words, in incremental adjustments to get as close to normal as is possible. The moodiness Catherine speaks of is not simply the straightforward expression of pain – as she says, she is not consciously aware of her pain at all times, although as we discussed this experience, we both spoke of how it is not complete unawareness, but more a 'background' sensation, an awareness that can be focused on, but can also be ignored. David described the background sensation of pain thus;

> *The best way I can describe it, it's like looking at a landscape, and sort of, using the body image as that landscape, whereas the chronic pain is more something – at the bottom of that lake rather than on that landscape, if that makes sense? It's almost a layer beneath that landscape, and I – it's difficult to sort of, to connect the one to the other – the layer behind that I can't quite perceive properly.*
>
> (David interview 1)

The experience of chronic pain is not easy to describe when it comes to the background sensation; once we focus on the pain long enough to begin to describe it, it is no longer a background sensation, instead it moves to the foreground of our awareness. In speaking of pain, we became more aware of it – as though by pointing it out, we were neither of us able to ignore our own pain.

A chronically painful body is an unreliable one; as Charlie observed:

> *You can't rely on your body to do what you want it to do any more, your confidence and your sense of control over your own life, it changes.*
>
> (Charlie, interview 1)

Pain destabilizes the self, but chronic pain results not in an unreliable body but a *reliably unreliable* body. While regaining some sense of control may be the aim of pain management treatment such as Julie spoke of, pushing patients to consider how to manage their energy and avoid situations that will lead to higher pain, there is also space for coming to terms with a body that is forever unreliable, a phenomenological self that is forever shattered asunder. This takes time; crip time is also the time taken to adjust to a reliably unreliable body.

When it comes to kink, the pain that results from play is reliable – it occurs in expected ways, in that it follows after activities that players know will cause pain, while chronic pain can spike after activities that are not associated with pain, and even after activities that have been performed without pain on previous occasions. In addition, the pain is likely to last for an expected amount of time – as acute pain, it contains the expectation that it will end. Thus, in playing with pain, participants are further adjusting to their reliably unreliable bodies, by re-establishing the reliability of non-chronic pain and re-confirming the unreliability of chronic pain, its abnormality. Kink pain in crip time is thus a part of their becoming disabled, their living with chronic pain.

Crip Time as Time to Become Crip

Living with chronic pain is, like for other disabled people, a part of identity and selfhood; participants all spoke of how living with chronic pain impacted their sense of self. Like disability, chronic pain interacts with other aspects of identity – and the conception of self narrated by participants is not fixed over time. Walden, in exploring the lives of lesbians living with chronic illness, states that a person's experience of illness, of fluctuating levels of pain and fatigue, "is a critical part of the process involved in integrating one's identity as a disabled/chronically ill lesbian into one's identity as an individual" (2009: 559); the same is no doubt true of people of other genders and/or sexualities, although the details of that process may be different. Edward, one of the older participants, explained that his sexual identity, as well as his erotic and sexual preferences, have changed over time, between and during relationships, and were impacted by how his disability and his age has altered his body. While Edward did not see these changes as the direct result of living with chronic pain or being disabled, he identified points where his experiences were affected by being disabled (such as his use of a wheelchair impacting his access to, and interaction with, social spaces), or by his pain specifically, on a practical and very embodied level (such as how pain affected his willingness to participate in submissive activities) and these experiences were a part of his sense of self.

For other participants, disability and living with chronic pain has impacted their sexuality directly. For some, this impact was not cast as either positive or negative; it simply *was* – this is exemplified by Charlie, who explained that because they acquired their disability as a young adult, they had not had long to establish their sense of sexual self;

> *I was only just becoming sexual before the [impairing event], so I hadn't fully explored my sexuality to any extent, so I can't separate out what my sexuality would have been without living with pain, in many ways. I mean, I didn't do [BDSM] before, except [laughs] the kinky kind of bondage stuff, as a kid, but I didn't seek it out – I suppose other sex was, more conventional non-kinky sex was satisfying, before the injury, so I think a lot of it was connected, uh, but I think I could have equally gone this was in an evolution of my sexuality anyway, so, and I think there must be an aspect of myself that was open to that in the first place, otherwise I wouldn't be doing* [BDSM].
>
> (Charlie, interview one)

For Charlie, becoming accustomed to their disability and chronic pain was experienced alongside their exploration of their sexual self, and thus they felt they could not say what they thought their sexuality would have been like had they remained non-disabled. This was not a particularly difficult question for Charlie to answer; they felt secure in their sexuality, and the time they had spent as a disabled person and living with chronic pain meant that they were, if not wholly happy with all aspects of their lives, at least accepting. Acceptance – and happiness – does not happen instantaneously, especially when living in diagnostic limbo can lead to a sense of being wrong, of disbelieving one's own self-knowledge (Wendell, 1996), and when living in a society that insists that disability is abnormal and unwanted. Crip time, therefore, includes not just time to live on an everyday level – the level of getting dressed or catching a bus – but on a longer timescale, that of a life lived; crip time includes the time needed to establish a positive disabled identity.

Julie, who experienced a great deal of change over the course of the 18 months over which the interviews occurred was less accepting than Charlie and Edward; she was still mourning the loss of her non-disabled and less painful past, as well as the possible futures of that earlier self. Kafer (2013) discusses futurity in relation to the specter of a disabled future in terms of non-disabled others looking at disabled children; crip time includes embracing a disabled future, in regarding a disabled future as wanted. However, embracing a disabled future is not always easy, even for disabled people; Julie is – and was – secure in her identity as a disabled woman, but a change in her impairment and the level of her everyday pain forced her to re-examine that identity.

> *In chronic pain management, they got to the point of wanky preaching about 'taking a step back, so the pain is still the same size but the perspective has shifted and so it seems less big and bad'… And after coping with a big life, with kink pain, chronic pain, interaction with others, work, fun, etc etc [sic], I've now got focussed [sic] on the illness side of things. In a way it never has been before. Some days all I see are my flat walls, and an hour of care from a carer. Others it's the same, but with added in paramedics. There's no space for kink in this life. Let alone kink pain. I'm not depressed, more just going through a period of mourning.*
>
> (Julie, diary entry)

This change, and the practical restrictions it put on her activities – particularly after discovering that orgasms carried a risk of minor stroke – was an emotional one for Julie, but one she was slowly beginning to adjust to; mourning her possible futures was a part of this, a part of her changing life, and a part of embracing her disabled future. Although Julie was still hoping for a change in her situation;

> *I'm clinging onto this being a temporary move rather than a permanent one. It can't get much worse so it has to get better. That's all that I've got left. In a way it's more positive than a few months back when I was mourning lost things, I've now lost so much I have to shift my mindset. Otherwise I'm just a woman in pyjamas in bed with the occasional filthy phonecall. I have to hold onto being more than that.*
>
> (Julie, interview 2)

This period of adjustment can be a mourning period, even when the person is already disabled, not just because it would be understood as a loss by non-disabled others, but because it is experienced as a loss by those who are adjusting; Julie has been restricted in terms of what she can do compared to her previous capacities, and her mourning – and frustration – is understandable, because she is no longer able to do something she wants to do. Acknowledging this mourning, giving time and space to become crip – to acknowledge and embrace oneself as disabled, as crip – is a part of crip time; this does not support the positioning of disability as negative, but instead leaves space to acknowledge that an unexpected change to the bodymind needs time to fully become a part of the phenomenological self.

Crip Time as Time to Adjust

In Charlie's words, in acquiring an impairment, or chronic pain:

> *There's lots of adjustment. I did lots of adjusting [with the leg injury], now I'm doing a lot more adjusting when the [diagnosis] got bad and now it's not getting better.*
>
> (Charlie, interview one)

Charlie's experience of pain has changed a great deal since their impairment event – not least because the original injury site is regarded as fully healed – and their more recent experience of increased fatigue and 'everyday' pain levels has led to further 'adjusting,' learning to once again live in a world that is systemically hostile to people living with pain and fatigue. Crip time therefore includes the time that individuals with acquired impairments – or progressive impairments – need to adjust, to reconstitute their self, within spaces of rehabilitation, but also outside of those spaces. In turning now to experiences of medicine and rehabilitation practices in this section, I do not intend to support a medical model approach to disability, or to support the medicalization of chronic pain, but to acknowledge that medical care is a part – to varying degrees – of the experience of living with chronic pain and disability (Kafer, 2013). Medicine has a huge impact on experiences of chronic pain, especially when some areas of disability explicitly exclude pain as an impairment, and also because treatment of pain is constructed as the responsibility of medicine.

Charlie observed that rehabilitation practices had changed a great deal since they became physically disabled, but although they found increasing attention was paid to 'whole-person' and holistic approaches to rehabilitation, it nonetheless took them several years to access particular services, particularly finding medics willing to discuss sexual function, for which they had to go to a different specialist department as the department who oversaw their care had no remit to consider sexuality, and felt unprepared to support them. This process of finding willing specialists – the process that Michelle described as "*going through the system*" (Michelle interview one) – takes time to access. The separation of specialists, and the time needed to access specialists, together with the experience of being passed from specialist to specialist for the treatment of seemingly distinct body parts, symptoms, or problems, may be holistic as far as medicine is concerned, but is experienced as a further separating out of the body, a further objectifying of the body (Illich, 1995; Young, 1997) – and a further removal of individuals' expertise and self-knowledge (Wendell, 1996). Furthermore, that access – and the amount of time needed to gain access – is unequal, not just in terms of geographic closeness to a hospital with the necessary specialists, but the willingness (and ability) of doctors to refer the particular individual to those specialists; this can be impacted by race, gender, and age, as well as the specific diagnosis or absence thereof. Rehabilitation time – what Frank (1995) calls the restitution narrative – is not smooth; some of the practices of rehabilitation are painful, as Michelle's narrative of undergoing 'corrective' surgery on her legs in her mid/late teens, that left her with greater pain, as well as changing her bodily shape and movement in ways she was neither accepting of or prepared for. In David's experience, some rehabilitation or pain management practices are boring (such as physiotherapy, or mindfulness), and there is a great deal of hit-and-miss approaches, trying different practices one after another in the hope of finding one that 'works,' or simply because there is a requirement to first try one practice in order to access the next. David found the practices of rehabilitation he was pushed toward had unwanted side effects that he struggled with; he found medication caused him to gain weight, which affected his self-image and self-confidence, and thus reconstituting his self with impairment was made more complicated.

This reconstitution of the self takes time – but it does not begin again every day, with every minor change in pain levels. It is only when there is a significant change – one that requires changes in the everyday and unremarkable practice of living – that the self must be reconstituted again. This is demonstrated by the change in Julie's narrative between her first and second interviews, where she spoke of once again learning to live with her disability when she lost the mobility of a wheelchair and became confined to her bed and her home, with greatly increased pain and fatigue;

> *My experience of myself now includes the pain centrally, and most of the time I am controlled by it rather than being able to control it. It dominates more than any dominating person of my choice can have hold over me. My chronic pain is far worse now than ever before, which knocks my confidence.*
>
> (Julie, interview two)

Julie's experience was very negative, and her narrative seemed initially quite bleak, but she was not the inarticulate non-human that previous theories of pain would have led the listener to believe. In many ways, telling the narrative of her experience was a part of Julie's rebuilding of herself; in speaking of her pain, she is able to claim her humanity through performing the role of a normal human – one who is able to speak of their pain, to describe it, to play with it, and to have that speaking and play listened to. A big part of Julie's narrative was that of her mourning the loss of her ability to take part in BDSM activities, especially as those activities had played a major role in her previous reconstitution, a few years previously, when she first became disabled. Kink helped Julie to stop seeing her chronic pain as something to 'overcome' or 'get over,' saying that:

> *At first [disability] made me more stubborn. I was going to prove it wrong and be a bigger, better me. Chronic pain was just a challenge to overcome. Since kink? This has allowed me to find a place to move away from the all encompassing pain/disability and just be me. Sure there are times when the chronic*

pain/disability have to play a part in the kink, I have major limitations, but to work beyond them is liberating. I've explored myself through the kink. Over the last few months I've lost a lot of confidence in my body as it has failed. My image of myself now includes my disability as a major component. I can't be the big and fun me any more, it's got lost in the pain for the time being. Having to hold onto to the hope I'll get "me" back.

(Julie, interview 2)

Julie found the space in kink to have time to grow accustomed to her new self, to embrace herself even though she was never particularly positive about being disabled, and without kink play, she was struggling – and was aware she was struggling – to readjust. However, this new unreliability was becoming reliably so; Julie was aware of the limitations of her body, and while her final interview was still tinged with loss, her sense of self came through more clearly, she was more confident in her reliably unreliable body.

Crip Time as Time to Manage Impairment

Pain management in an unreliable body is not a straightforward matter; the intervals of time between medications can stretch and contort, pain may make sleep impossible, or sleep the only activity possible, and a carefully established routine can be broken by an unforeseen, unplanned-for event. A day can last forever and also be slept away. Pre-resting to prepare for an event – forcing yourself to do even less in the hope of making more energy available the next day and avoiding pain-inducing activity – can be necessary even though it may prove useless, and a flare-up result anyway. As Natalie described it, while activity could reliably result in increased fatigue and pain, resting was not so reliable. Recovery from a spike in pain or fatigue could take days, or weeks, or months[1]; kink almost always resulted in higher pain and fatigue, but was judged worth it.

For all the participants, pain levels were not constant; Edward described his pain as intermittent rather than chronic, and the rest all reported that sometimes they experienced more pain, sometimes less. There tends to be an assumption that chronic pain is constant, in terms of both intensity and duration, this is not necessarily the case, and while Edward preferred the term intermittent because he had long pain-free periods, his diagnosis is such that his pain could also be understood as chronic, which he acknowledged. Medication helped sometimes, as did a host of other pain management techniques, from yoga to acupuncture; most of the participants used multiple management techniques together, as well as multiple medications, in order to increase the time, they spent in less pain, or to live with that pain. For Charlie, kink formed a part of their pain management; they reported that

In any sort of kink or sex kind of play … sometimes I've been able to, uh, extend the period between using analgesia because of the impact of the endorphins, and just, whatever.

(Charlie, interview one)

For all the participants, kink was not only pleasurable, but produced a temporary relief from pain, in that they felt less pain, the quality of their pain changed, or they were focused elsewhere; I will turn to the control of pain at a later point but for the moment it is the relationship between time and the participants' experience of their pain that is my focus. Within the context of crip time, then, managing pain requires time – requires time to engage in pain control methods. One of these methods, particularly for those who live with chronic pain and fatigue, is pacing – carefully measuring out time and energy in order to complete tasks without resulting in pain or fatigue flare-ups.

Crip Time as Pacing

When it comes to living with chronic pain, which is so often accompanied by fatigue, a great deal of emphasis is placed on 'pacing' yourself as a form of pain management – especially in rehabilitation settings – and the need to 'manage' time and lower-pain days so as not to provoke periods of increased pain or fatigue. While pacing is useful, it is also frustrating, irritating, and runs counter to the ideal of achievement; as Catherine put it:

> *Oh yes, pacing. I'm relatively good at pacing, practically speaking. Emotionally it kills me – especially while I've got a lot to do, like right now. If I have a list of tasks and have to go to bed, I get REALLY angry with myself. Like 'what are you even for?' angry. But practically speaking I can do it, and I know I have to.*
>
> (Catherine, interview 2)

However, pacing also opens up the individual to victim-blaming discourses, where a failure to properly perform pacing is a failure of proper self-care, a failure to use the full "range of market commodities that hold out the promise of therapeutic interventions into the relative failures of physical, cognitive and affective embodiment" (Shildrick, 2015: 11) offered by neoliberal society. Those who practice pacing, who attempt to manage pain by managing their time, are caught between a rock and a hard place; the demands of keeping up with the pace of life require pacing, but those demands are such that they will never be properly met, as neoliberalism keeps bodies as always debilitated in order to sustain profit and markets (Mitchell and Snyder, 2015; Shildrick, 2015). At the same time, if pacing is not seen to be properly performed – or even if it is – and it (inevitably) fails to adequately prevent pain or fatigue, it is the *individual* that is marked as a failure, and the pace of life is not questioned. Crip pacing, therefore, is not just about self-management to optimize production, but self-management to optimize *joy*, to take care of oneself and pleasure in that care; crip pacing as a form of politicized self-care (Ahmed, 2014).

As Siebers (2008) points out, passing as normal is exhausting; for participants who live with fatigue or limited as well as chronic pain, passing as normal can only be sustained for so long, if at all. David finds his pain and fatigue impacts every aspect of his life, and when it comes to his kink play, he knows that playing for longer periods of time, or maintaining certain positions, or movements, is difficult, and this requires him to explain to and negotiate with his partners – such as needing to change position, or to only use certain equipment. It is this performance of disability – of making pain and fatigue visible – that is undesirable, that desexualizes him, and thus is risky for David, opening him up to abjection and being repositioned as less-than-able, and thus less-than-human.

Julie, on the other hand, finds a certain freedom in living with fatigue and pain, saying:

> *I only have limited energy and stuff with the pain, so I have to – I get the choice. It's quite liberating in some circumstances, I find, cos I now have to choose what I do and don't do, I can't just do everything, uh, because I've got these limiting pains, so I – I do appreciate all those choices I make.*
>
> (Julie, interview one)

In being forced to make choices – sometimes difficult choices, as Natalie's narrative of missing such socially-significant events as funerals and weddings showed – due to a mismatch between the pace of life and the restrictions of an ill and painful body, Julie and Natalie are made disabled, pushed to live as abnormal. However, their sense of liberation shows that matching the pace of life demanded by ableist social structures is not necessarily rewarding in itself; there is no inherent joy in being normal, while being abnormal can be (or can be made to be) freeing and joyous. This joy in rejecting a normative pace of life (even if the rejection is the consequence of a loss of capacity) demonstrates the joy that can be found in living crip, in crip ways of moving through time.

Natalie spoke of her need to weigh the energy costs of each activity – asking herself firstly if she has the energy to do the activity in the first place, and secondly if the resulting pain and fatigue will be worth both the loss of energy *and* the resulting pain and fatigue the activity will inevitably cause. While this may seem like a simple cost-benefit analysis – the risks of an action against the risks of not doing it – there is great pressure to *do*, to meet the pace of life and activity level demanded by normative society; it is not acceptable to only do some of the task (some of the shopping, part of the wedding), or to admit that the reason for not doing any of the activity is that while you may be able to right that moment, you have decided it will not be worth the pain or the fatigue that will result, even if the resulting fatigue will impact your ability to complete other activities. This is because the admission of pain and fatigue is a reminder that they are abnormal, forcing the listener to face not just the pain of the speaker, but also the possibility of their own pain. Speaking of pain and fatigue also forces the person in pain to confront their pain again – to acknowledge that pain is a part of their lives, that they live an abnormal life; it is this discomfort that Julie showed when admitting she rarely told others she lives with chronic pain.

For Charlie, who has lived with chronic pain and fatigue for many years, but had more recently experienced an increase in fatigue, the endurance aspect of their BDSM play particularly appealed to them, as a counter to experiences and sensations of hardship. I also interpreted Charlie's narrative of the appeal of 'enduring' through kink as to include countering the sensation of fatigue, a way of speaking back to fatigue. Charlie, however, felt it was more about experiences of trauma and hardship than fatigue – feeling that instead fatigue limits their capability to endure – and was only about fatigue on a very limited level. I wish to draw attention to the differences in understanding here as it highlights how multiple readings can be found in the same narrative; it is perhaps my own experience of fatigue that has affected my reading of Charlie's narrative, and assigning greater importance to fatigue than they have done. I wish to acknowledge this difference, but also concede to Charlie – and thus emphasize that the endurance aspects of some forms of BDSM play (flogging, but also bondage, in particular) played a role in Charlie's integration of their experience of hardship and trauma into their self.

Running parallel to Charlie's narrative of why they consciously choose to engage in play, Natalie's narrative showed that it is also difficult to acknowledge when she has decided that a particular activity (not just sex or play) is worth the pain and fatigue – and particularly so when the activity could be deemed 'frivolous' or even selfish by an observer, such as when the activity serves no function beyond the pleasure of Natalie (and her husband). For Natalie, kink served as a reward, as a celebration of periods when she felt herself capable of enduring, of being strong – as well as something to look forward to in the times when she and her husband both felt unable to do what they wanted to do; she explained that:

> *When we're both in poor physical shape and can't do much, we talk about all the things we'll do when we're better.*
>
> (Natalie, interview 1)

David also saw that time when he was not capable of engaging in kink play as potentially useful;

> *At the same time, a case of roll with it, figure what is possible; sort of make use of the time to connect in other ways. Talk. Bounce ideas backwards and forwards. Just making time can be a… it's not wasted time.*
>
> (David, interview two)

This 'useful' downtime, a time to talk and reassess – however playfully – is a part of crip time, a part of its ebbing and flowing, and can be fought against or it can be gone with; it can be accepted, or rejected. Pacing as an act of self-care can require going with the flow, but can also take the form of fighting back, refusing to go with the flow, even though this makes the body less reliable, increases the chances of a flare.

Crip Time as Time to Think and Do Slowly

A flare in chronic pain can often be accompanied by other changes in the capacities of the bodymind. When my own pain flares, I am more tired, my balance and sense of bodily orientation in space is altered – I fall more easily, struggle to judge distances or hold objects – and my cognitive abilities are limited, I struggle to communicate, or to understand. Cognition may not, at first, seem dependent on time, but there is space to consider how people with cognitive impairments and people with learning disabilities are often described as 'slow' – slow readers, slow to meet developmental targets, slow to understand. As Chen describes it, writing through the concept of crip cognition:

> maybe we can talk about an expected temporal trajectory, not consistent throughout but—like sexual development narratives—having its own proper spurts and ebbs, a mapped journey of cognitive elaboration (known to cognitive scientists and pediatricians as development), such that a cognitive identity can be felt and affirmed in a way that produces the effect of a 'cis' [cognitive ability].
> (Chen, 2014: 178)

Those of us with unexpected trajectories and abnormal cognitive abilities are something queer, something crip. This acknowledgment of non-normative cognitive identities – as distinct from both cognitive 'normality' and the neuroatypicality identified by autistic individuals (which itself may be considered to overlap with crip cognition) is reliant on the understanding that "an information-handling reading of cognition, rather than being a remote disciplinary feature proper only to cognitive science, is integral to the prevailing mechanisms for the contemporary production of knowledge" (2014: 178); ableism is expressed in a preference for normative *thinking* as well as normative ways of doing and being.

For the participants, pain and fatigue was sometimes accompanied by 'brain fog,' a state of thinking slowly, of a fogged-up brain, of a loss of cognitive faculties akin to having one's brain replaced by marshmallows and where following a thought is like wading through treacle. For Natalie, the cognitive symptoms of impairment "killed [her sexuality] dead" (Natalie, interview 2); she reported feeling very few, if any, sexual feelings, experienced no sexual desire – and as a result did not feel any particular sexual identity. For other participants, brain fog impacted their sense of self, not as pain did – brain fog being temporary, while pain was a constant (if fluctuating) experience – with temporary loss of faculties leading to their frustration with themselves, and awareness that they frustrated others with their inability to communicate easily or grasp basic facts. For Catherine, this was in addition to the more everyday effects of her neuro-atypical cognition.

Conclusion

In thinking slowing – in moving and being slow – crip ways of living with pain and fatigue contrast most strongly with normative pace of life demands. And making space for this deliberate – and necessary – slowness becomes important – even if that space-making isn't wanted so much as needed. Making space for slowness and pacing, and rejecting them in favor of speed and activity, thus becomes about control. Which is where we turn next.

Note

1 Or never happen at all.

References

Ahmed S (2006) *Queer Phenomenology: Orientations, Objects, Others*. London: Duke University Press.

Ahmed S (2014) Selfcare as Warfare. Available at: http://feministkilljoys.com/2014/08/25/selfcare-as-warfare/ (accessed 29 May 2015).

Chen MY (2014) Brain Fog: The Race for Cripistemology. *Journal of Literary & Cultural Disability Studies* 8(2): 171–184. DOI: 10.1353/jlc.2014.0015.

Conrad P and Muñoz VL (2010) The Medicalization of Chronic Pain. *Tidsskrift for Forskning: Sygdom og Samfund* 13: 13–25. DOI: 10.7146/tfss.v7i13.4147.

Crary J (2013) *24/7: Late Capitalism and the Ends of Sleep*. London: Verso.

Edelman L (2004) *No Future: Queer Theory and the Death Drive*. Durham, NC: Duke University Press.

Foucault M (1973) *The Birth of the Clinic: An Archaeology of Medical Perception* (trans. AM Sheridan). London: Tavistock Publications Ltd.

Frank AW (1995) *The Wounded Storyteller*. Chicago, IL: University of Chicago Press.

Goodley D (2014) *Dis/Ability Studies: Theorising Disablism and Ableism*. Abingdon: Routledge.

Halberstam J (2005) *In a Queer Time and Place: Transgender Bodies, Subcultural Lives*. New York: New York University Press.

Hickey-Moody A (2015) Slow Life and Ecologies of Sensation. *Feminist Review* 111: 140–148. DOI: 10.1057/fr.2015.40.

Illich I (1995) *Limits to Medicine: Medical Nemesis, the Expropriation of Health*. London: Marion Boyars Publishers Ltd.

Inckle K (2015) Debilitating times: compulsory Ablebodiedness and White Privilege in Theory and Practice. *Feminist Review* 111: 42–58. DOI: 10.1057/fr.2015.38.

Jain SL (2013) *Malignant: How Cancer Becomes Us*. Oakland: University of California Press.

Kafer A (2013) *Feminist, Queer, Crip*. Bloomington and Indianapolis: Indiana University Press.

Kumari Campbell F (2009) *Contours of Ableism: The Production of Disability and Abledness*. Basingstoke: Palgrave Macmillan.

McRuer R (2006) *Crip Theory: Cultural Signs of Queerness and Disability*. New York: NYU Press.

Mitchell DT and Snyder SL (2015) *The Biopolitics of Disability: Neoliberalism, Ablenationalism, and Peripheral Embodiment*. Ann Arbour: University of Michigan Press.

Price M (2015) The Bodymind Problem and the Possibilities of Pain. *Hypatia* 30(1): 268–284. DOI: 10.1111/hypa.12127.

Puar JK (2009) Prognosis Time: Towards a Geopolictics of Affect, Debility and Capacity. *Women and Performance: A Journal of Feminist Theory* 19(2): 161–172.

Rogers C (2009) (S)excerpts from a Life Told: Sex, Gender and Learning Disability. *Sexualities* 12(3): 270–288.

Shildrick M (2015) Living on; Not Getting Better. *Feminist Review* 111: 10–24. DOI: 10.1057/fr.2015.22.

Siebers T (2008) *Disability Theory*. Ann Arbour: University of Michigan Press.

Tyler I (2013) *Revolting Subjects: Social Abjection and Resistance in Neoliberal Britain*. London: Zed Books.

Walden EJ (2009) An Exploration of the Experience of Lesbians with Chronic Illness. *Journal of Homosexuality* 56(5): 548–574.

Wearing S, Gunaratnam Y and Gedalof I (2015) Frailty and Debility. *Feminist Review* 111: 1–9. DOI: 10.1057/fr.2015.39.

Wendell S (1996) *The Rejected Body: Feminist Philosophical Reflections on Disability*. New York: Routledge.

Young K (1997) *Presence in the Flesh: The Body in Medicine*. Cambridge, MA: Harvard University Press.

5 Controlled/Uncontrolled

Choosing terminology in this section was not easy; there was no single phrase that jumped out at me. Participants spoke of 'managing' pain, of 'coping with' pain, fatigue or frustration, and spoke of feeling as though pain 'controlled' their lives. I went with control because it felt closest to what I heard and felt; the need to make conscious decisions about how to interact with their pain, the need to feel connected to their bodymind, the need to perform in expected ways in order to access care. There is possibly another word that would encapsulate all this better, but neither my participants nor I could find one. So, in choosing 'control' I am deliberately drawing a line in this chapter between these actions (and inactions) and deeper social and cultural expectations around self-control and containment, and the 'civilized' able bodymind.

Stigma and Abjection

Stigma is cast upon us due to "an undesired differentness from what [others] had expected" (Goffman, 2006: 132); in the case of disabled people, that differentness is from the expected norms in terms of appearance, configuration, and/or capacity of the bodymind. To follow Goffman, disabled people can either live with stigma, try to cure their difference, or overcome stigma through excelling in some other area, such as sporting prowess; rather than disagree with Goffman, I want to dig deeper in the twin roles of stigma and abjection in the lives of my participants and people living with chronic pain more broadly. In the case of disability, stigma is closely tied to abjection, which, in Kristeva's words, is a challenge to order – "it is thus not lack of cleanliness or health that causes abjection but what disturbs identity, system, order. What does not respect borders, positions, rules. The in-between, the ambiguous, the composite" (1997: 232). Abjection requires containment in certain bodies, in the bodies of certain others (McRuer, 2006), and it creates spaces and zones of exclusion (Tyler, 2013) – both physically (in terms of inaccessible spaces and segregated education) but also in a wider discourse of 'them' and 'us,' of othering.

Stigmatized bodies are those which are repulsive, disgusting, abject – due to a fear of disability, a horror of bodily difference (McRuer, 2006; Shildrick, 2009) the discursively normal subject expresses this disgust, this abjection, as a "response to

DOI: 10.4324/9781003006237-6

that stuff which threatens to overwhelm their body border and their attempts to turn away and distance themselves" (Tyler, 2013: 27). Disgust, as Miller (Miller, 1997) points out, is often intertwined with fear, particularly fear of contamination, or fear of the possibility that the disgusted person could themselves become disgusting, become stigmatized through acquiring disability. Thus, stigmatized disabled bodyminds are horrifying and repulsive because they act as reminders of the fragility of normality – of how close the normal human is to being abnormal, or to being lesser (ibid., 1997); as Hughes writes, "at an existential level the presence of the disabled body is unsettling for non-disabled people who are often in denial about their own vulnerability. This is the psychological and emotional component of … ableism" (Hughes, 2012: 18). This existential unsettling can also be named as *ontological impossibility* – an inability to perceive of a future possibility (or, if we are honest about aging: future inevitability) of becoming disabled, of living while disabled.

Bodyminds that wobble, that leak (Liddiard and Slater, 2017), that are missing parts or with parts that don't work, that shout at the wrong time and twitch and mutter are all disabled bodyminds – and all are responded to with fear, disgust, and staring (Garland-Thomson, 2009). Given that

> abjection links the lived experience of the body, the socially and culturally specific meanings of the body, the cultural investment in selectively marking the body, the privileging of some parts and the functions while resolutely minimizing or leaving un- or underrepresented other parts or functions.
>
> (Grosz, 1994: 192)

and as Kumari Campbell observes, "cultural practices of shaping bodies can affect the etiology of 'typical' human functioning" (Kumari Campbell, 2009b: 18), normality is thus culturally constituted and constructed, continually being made and continually shifting in its demands; the normal bodymind is one that has all the expected parts in working order, that speaks at the right time and volume, and moves in expected ways – that is not just whole but *controlled* and civilized in their wholeness. For the non-disabled, there is a continual anxious need to perform cleanliness and wholeness (Miller, 1997; Tyler, 2013), to perform able-bodymindedness and demonstrate that one is not the abject; Kristeva's clean and proper body (1997) is Hughes' normative one (2012), and for Tyler (2013), abjection is contingent on expressions of normativity – on being controlled in a civilized way.

There is a moral judgment against failure to perform this expected civilization (Miller, 1997), to perform normativity (Hughes, 2012), and thus a moral judgment against being disabled, against receiving welfare, against needing assistance and failing to be properly independent (Tyler, 2013; Wendell, 1996). Disabled people, along with migrants, people of color, and benefits claimants are national abjects, in ways that are different and the same, as "ideological conductors [are] mobilized to do the dirty work of neoliberal governmentality. They are symbolic and material scapegoats, the mediating agencies through which the social decomposition effected by market deregulation and welfare retrenchment are legitimized" (Tyler, 2013: 9). Importance is therefore placed on passing as normal, as non-disabled – as properly rehabilitated and not at fault – precisely because "passing is not just about the impaired person hiding their impairment or morphing their disability … [it] is about keeping the colonizer happy by not disturbing the peace, containing the matter that is potentially out of place" (Kumari Campbell, 2009b: 44). However, as Tyler (2013) observes, national abjects remain at the center of public life even when they attempt to pass as normal, because they must be seen in order to be controlled; the threat of abjection is no threat without the visible abject. They are what Braidotti terms 'disposable' bodies, who "experience dispossession of their embodied and embedded selves, in a political economy of repeated and structurally enforced eviction" (2011: 6).

In abjection, disability is a failure of a properly-controlled body, a failure of self-control (McRuer, 2006), and an object of moral disgust, where "a physical experience of disgust slides into contempt and judgments of value. Yet because disgust is an emotion associated with involuntary bodily reaction, moral disgust is often experienced, or retroactively understood, as a natural response" (Tyler, 2013: 22–23). It is this appearance of naturalness that ableism relies on in the system of compulsory able-bodymindedness. Within this, bodies must be civilized – must be controlled according to social norms (Miller, 1997; Williams and Bendelow, 1998); the sick body must be disciplined (de Wolfe, 2002), and doubt is cast on bodies that are not controlled. The risk/danger discourses of contagion, of the abject catching like disease, which lead to what Williams and Bendelow (1998) call 'surveillance medicine,' identifying precursors of future illness or impairment feed into processes of abjection as

> individuals are advised, cajoled and encouraged by health promoters to assess critically their risks of succumbing to disease and to change their behaviors accordingly. In doing so, a 'victim-blaming ideology' develops – one in which individuals are instructed to take responsibility for their health at a time when they are least able to do so.
>
> (ibid., 1998: 71)

Tying in with the hyper-individualizing discourses of responsibility and meritocracy in neoliberalism, the individual holds responsibility of their health, success, achievement, and so on, effectively depoliticizing disability, and thus disability is "presented as a fact of life requiring determination and courage, not as a system marking some bodies, some ways of thinking, and patterns of movement as deviant and unworthy" (Kafer, 2013: 89); failure to perform, to be normal, to be independent and controlled and to perform taking control and engaging in rehabilitation, marks one as morally disgusting, as abject, as stigmatized – and therefore disability is "ontologically invalid or 'uncivilized'" (Hughes, 2012: 18), and rehabilitation must cure or kill.

A controlled and controllable body, is also a docile, plastic, and moldable object, composed of individual parts that are either fixable or replaceable (Grosz, 1994; Williams and Bendelow, 1998). At the same time,

> The line between normality and deviance is no longer rigid, or regarded as naturally given; it is shifting and variable… In today's 'normalization society', normality is no longer considered an immutable, permanent fact of the matter; instead, it is seen as a challenge, as something that can be designed and produced, as a phenomenon that changes with time. Normality is no longer an external constraint that society imposes on its members; it is formed and shaped by acting subjects themselves. The conception of normality that currently prevails could be termed flexible-normalistic.
>
> (Waldschmidt, 2005: 191–192)

As a result, normality is both compulsory and an idealistic conception; we can never achieve perfect normality, because it constantly shifts beyond reach of the individual; we exist in a state of anxiety over our own lack of normality. The neoliberal self-policing subject, in seeking normality, internalizes their anxiety.

This anxiety to be normal – to not become abject, to distance ourselves from the abject – includes an emphasis on *being healthy* – on being in control of one's self, on having a self-disciplined body. As "health is the accumulative expression of how we 'matter' in our social worlds" (Adelson, 2010: 50–51), there is a moral dimension to health, where ill health, and even the apparent failure to perform control of one's health, becomes a personal failure of self-control, and of needing another (the doctor) to control one's body, rather than simply advising on *how* to control it; this echoes the moral dimension of the asylum discourse,[1] where immorality was equated with disability, a lack of civilization, and queerness. Wendell writes of how her illness, ME/CFS,

> was for a while described in the media primarily in terms of the symbolic meanings that were created for it in the mid-1980s; it was the 'yuppie flu', a punishment of nature visited upon the ambitious, especially ambitious women… the mythic descriptions are more exciting and more reassuring to the healthy than the reality.
>
> (1996: 62)

This reassurance is important, tied as it is to a victim-blaming approach that says, in effect, 'I didn't do/am not doing *that*, so bad things will not happen to me.'

As a part of controlling our bodily selves – which, it should be noted, includes our mental health – we must assess our own risks of contracting illness and change our lifestyles in order to minimize this risk; as already mentioned, this results in a discourse that blames the sick person for becoming ill (Williams and Bendelow, 1998).[2] The risk and moral danger discourses that intertwine with discourses of health are

> Articulated and expressed… through public health campaigns and the forms of 'surveillance medicine' they spawn… risks to health are no longer conceptualized in existing places and spaces, nor in terms of personal hygiene. Instead, the contemporary emphasis on health promotion, lifestyles and the 'green response' to ecological dangers has meant that risks are located everywhere.
>
> (Williams and Bendelow, 1998: 70–71)

As a result, we must be ever-vigilant to existing risk and flexible enough to change when new risks are identified by the appropriate, knowledgeable, authorities. At this point, it is relevant to note that 'being healthy' is firmly tied to ideals of food consumption and exercise – which is tied to class and income through access to alternative 'healthy' options,[3] echoing and intertwined with discourses of obesity and the moral panic over weight (Cooper, 2010; Gordon, 2020).

In discourses of 'being healthy,' which Tremain (2005) identifies as one of the multiple forms of governmentality, it is easy to see how the body has itself become a fetishized commodity, with

> Lifestyle and body planning… [forming] a normal part of life in post-traditional, reflexive environments. What might at first appear to be a wholesale movement towards the cultivation of bodily appearance is… on closer inspection, an expression of a much deeper underlying concern to actively control and 'construct' the body through a pluralization of lifestyle options and choices that reflexive modernity makes possible.
>
> (Williams and Bendelow, 1998: 74)

Having the 'right attitude' toward health and fitness is paralleled by the cosmetic surgery industry; being normal – or striving for normality – requires people to perform fitness (or, as McRuer (2006) puts it, athleticism) and health, while being disabled, chronically ill, or in pain can often form major barriers to performing health from the outset. The tendency to refer to such acts of performing health and fitness as self-care, and hence framing them in terms of an individual and depoliticized act,[4] which enables those of us worn down by neoliberalism, capitalism, racism, sexism, and/or ableism, and so on to get back up and carry on working, ignores that such performances of conspicuous health may, for disabled people or those with impairments, present instead as *work*, or be inaccessible.

Aside from issues of financial resources and environmental accessibility, for many chronically ill and disabled people, the act of self-care itself becomes more complex – either through the need for assistance for basic personal care, or through the simple fact that some people simply require more time[5] and planning to carry out such tasks (Kafer, 2013; Wendell, 1996); "for those who live with chronic fatigue or pain, for example, the present moment must often be measured against the moment to come" (Kafer, 2013: 39). The need to perform self-care through conspicuous health – through acts of exercise and 'healthy' food consumption, rather than watching children's cartoons and eating chocolate[6] – presents a further barrier; there is an increasing need for acts of self-care to be recognizable as such to non-disabled others, in order to be acknowledged as such. At the same time as such barriers are being thrown up, the figure of the athletic super-crip forms another, spectral, barrier – the disabled figure who has 'overcome' their disability through becoming exceptionally good at a particular sport, or completed a particular event, from becoming a Paralympic athlete to climbing Everest (Kafer, 2013; Sumpter, 2012; Young, 2012); the continual message received by chronically ill people and those with mental health or cognitive impairment diagnoses (in particular) is that with the 'right' diet, exercise, or vitamin supplement – along with the right attitude – they will be 'cured,' while their more obviously and visibly disabled peers will be able to overcome their impairments.

Theorizing understandings of control enables further links to be drawn between social expectations of a normal bodymind – in terms of comportment, containment, and capacities – and crip uses and contestations of control. The uses of control by participants are an important consideration – control is not easily divided into normal and abnormal, into control and lack thereof, and nor should it be; as participants showed, they contested demands for control even as they sought out control – and sought spaces to be uncontrolled through other forms of control. Their consecratory and complicated narratives of control often conflicted, but nonetheless control played an important part in participants' narratives of chronic pain, particularly in terms of controlling pain – both in an attempt to perform proper humanity, but also in an attempt to re-establish their phenomenological self in the face of an unreliable bodymind. I want to move onwards with a quote from Julie, who explained how she felt about controlling her chronic pain:

> *Controlling pain is important. Whether that be resting to decrease some pain, using painkillers if they work, moving position at the simplest level. Kink is taking this to its natural conclusion by making pain to control.*
>
> (Julie, interview 2)

Sex and Control

The control of emotions is a part of self-control, whether those emotions are understood as positive or negative by observers; controlling emotional responses to experiences of pain, disability, and chronic illness is a necessary part of performing proper bodymindedness, particularly for disabled people and people living with chronic pain. Controlling emotion does not mean expressing little emotion, but performing *proper* emotion, or expressing emotion in appropriate ways. This is exemplified by how children learn to react appropriately to acute pain incidents – for example, when a small child, still learning to walk, falls in the process of play and scrapes a knee, their tears and vocal cries are accepted as a 'normal' reaction by other small children and adults, although their parent may seek to quieten their response with cuddles and fussing over their injury. However, when an older child falls during play, they may well try to hold back tears, to 'get over it' quickly and continue their game, not seeking out a parent's attention; a child who fails to contain their reaction may be mocked by others as being a 'big baby,' and if that child is a boy, he may be told to 'man up,' or another phrase implying that expressions of hurt are feminizing as well as improper. To say that the smaller child feels *more pain* is to do an injustice to the older; the older child may well have felt like bawling and demanding that somebody kiss their knee better, but they have learnt that it is not appropriate behavior. Proper bodymindedness requires proper emotional control.

Living with chronic pain requires emotional control – but for participants, it was also an emotional experience, not just in terms of sadness or crying out with pain (although there is plenty of that). Catherine spoke of expressing her pain as irritability, anger, and depression – experiencing depression in particular is common among those living with chronic pain (Nielsen and Fernandez, 2010; Thomas and Johnson, 2000), and those living with chronic pain are frequently prescribed antidepressants along with analgesics.[7] However, there are proper and improper spaces and times in which the emotions of pain can be expressed, as well as proper audiences; expressing pain and weakness is a private act when it is acceptable at all. For the participants, finding times and spaces to express emotional responses to pain – as well as a receptive audience – was one of the pleasures of BDSM, which provided a space for engaging with bodies and emotions. This is not to say that BDSM is free of control – or *out of control* – but that the rules of behavior in play make space for emotions, for screaming and crying and seeking comforting touch. The expression of emotion is encouraged, even required.

As chronic pain is expected to be – and very frequently is – emotionally negative, as living with chronic pain can lead to a negative perception of the bodily self – especially a body that is unreliable, and so frequently the object of others' abjection. This only becomes increased when the person living with chronic pain must restrict the expression of their emotional response to their chronic pain, limiting what they express, where they express those feelings, and who is present when they do. Many participants spoke of feeling pressured to remain silent and limit how much, and to who, they expressed emotional responses to their chronic pain, and this did sometimes include when interacting with play partners – as focusing too much on their chronic pain would make them less attractive as a play partner. Charlie explained that they kept explanations of chronic pain to a minimum, focusing on the practical aspects – such as where they could not be flogged – unless they were playing with a close friend, or someone who also lived with chronic pain. This practical, quantitative, emotionless evaluation of pain was something participants mentioned performing for medics and care providers, particularly in cases where they felt an emotional response would not help them access medication or care – for fear of being labeled drug-seeking, hysterical, or exaggerating. This tactical performance of pain, while sometimes useful, cut both ways; Charlie and Catherine both felt that being unemotional about their pain meant listeners could be less sympathetic – and less inclined to provide medication – but that being perceived as too emotional meant that they were less likely to be believed. Expressing emotional responses to pain was a minefield for all the participants, and one that they all negotiated carefully.

However, in using pain within their play, participants were able to engage emotionally with their pain, and with their bodily selves, in a controlled space, and in ways in which they were in control, rather than relying on the judgment of medics or caregivers, as Julie explained;

> *It's about controlling my body, or allowing someone else to control it, in certain ways.*
>
> (Julie, interview 1)

The act of receiving pain was a way to connect with the somatic sensation of pain, and express emotional responses, but an activity they could call a stop to – as well as an experience of pain they know will end. Julie explained that when it came to chronic pain,

> *[she deals] with not dealing with it.... And so, then the, um, the kind of kink pain is kind of dealing with it and kind of exploring through that ... so it's not shutting it all out as far as I can, it's actually experiencing it.*
>
> (Julie, interview 1)

This control of the experience of pain, and the space to be uncontrolled in their response to pain, can be read as the opposite to living with chronic pain – with chronic pain as an experience that they did not choose to have, and that they cannot put an end to, but nonetheless are required to be controlled in their response to – and thus is a space to speak back to the pain. For Natalie, BDSM play turns her menacing chronic pain into something else, something she is able to experience as painful but also positive, and she sees this as a conscious subverting of her experience of chronic pain through BDSM play; in this way sex and play is, for her, an act of reclaiming the self, and of creating a space of emotional response. Julie found that BDSM play provided her with a space to re-engage positively with her bodily self;

> *[BDSM] has allowed [her] to find a place to move away from the all encompassing pain/disability and just be [herself].*
>
> (Julie, interview two)

This 'being herself' comes complete with expression of emotion – a space where Julie is not pressured to be pain-free, or to perform disability. Julie did not start practicing BDSM until after she first came to live with chronic pain, and her interest in play pain and submission developed alongside her new identity as a person living with chronic pain. She feels that, through BDSM, she is

> *Starting to understand [her] body beyond the pain, beyond the chronic pain ... beyond the pain even if it's been induced even in a kink-type setting.*
>
> (Julie, interview two)

This understanding of the self, of the bodymind can only come with expression of emotion, with space to fully feel, and BDSM gives Julie a positive experience of pain, and of her body, even with chronic pain, which she had experienced, and continues to experience, as overwhelmingly negative.

All the participants placed importance on their ability to control their pain, and in ways they chose. BDSM provided some of the participants with a way to control their chronic pain, through creating increased pain, which will be stopped at any point in the near future, and that they can both plan for and control – through discussion with their play partner, and through calling a stop to the scene. Catherine explained that exploring what she gets pleasure from, or not, is important;

> *I can try something, rather than having it sort of imposed on me that this is the situation. And I can find out if it's a type of pain that I like or not. So, some things are not a sort of pain I enjoy.*
>
> (Catherine, interview one)

In Julie's words;

> *I think, um, I like it because it's being in control of the pain. Or there's a level of, yeah, I'm in control rather than my body being in control. Even though my body then reacts to the pain in certain ways. But it's that I'm deciding to have pain, rather than it deciding to have me, type stuff.*
>
> (Julie, interview 1)

Pain and Control

To return to ideas of pain discussed in the first chapter, if we take the understanding of pain as an attack on the phenomenological self (Langdridge, 2007; Scarry, 1985), and that therefore the experience of pain requires a remake of the world and of the self, we then need to consider how the world and the self is remade within chronic pain. If we take the assumption that chronic pain works on the phenomenological self like acute pain, along normative lines, it requires the person living with chronic pain to have the world and the self constantly broken and remade. I would argue, however, based on the narratives of the participants, that chronic pain is experienced differently to acute pain – it is not experienced as externally-caused, imposed from outside the self, and once pain is established as chronic, it has no expectation of stopping in the near future; the pain must be lived with. Chronic pain does not require constant remaking of the world and of the self because it becomes the new state of being; one becomes a person who lives with pain rather than a person, or body in pain. The normative reading of pain does not fully grasp this, pain is not supposed to be normal because understandings of pain are that it is acute, that it will pass in time.

For my participants, it was impossible to maintain a state of inarticulate, dishuman distress for very long, although periods of high pain are often experienced as exactly that – periods when pain becomes all that can be experienced;

> *You might have to close off because of pain, because that's all you can deal with, but at times where it's sort of moderate to background, you can engage with it in different ways, it's not shutting you down in the same way. There's times when it's just too extreme, you just have to shut down, take yourself away, and those are the times you don't do anything with anybody.*
>
> (Charlie, interview 2)

But afterwards, once the period of high pain has ceased – even when pain is still experienced – they desired to find the self once more, to counteract pain and to re-establish their selfhood and everyday (in)activities – more simply, to actively live. When chronic pain changes in the long-term (rather than day-to-day fluctuations), it is not quite a new experience of pain, as the person is already living with chronic pain; they have already experienced what it is to remake the self – as demonstrated by Charlie's recent, and Julie's ongoing, changes in pain types and levels. Julie's impairment is progressive – it is expected to get worse in time – and as she explains,

> *Loss of control is a big part of disability when it is a progressive condition like mine. I've slowly had to give up things that I thought were important or vital to life (even if I now think of them as solely distant memories and nothing particularly important). I try to "just accept" as stressing about what I'm not doing doesn't help me feel any better in this moment in time.*
>
> (Julie, interview 2)

Catherine and Julie explained that they found that, over time, their chronic pain has not lessened, but it draws less of their focus; they are able to continue on (as indeed they must), and the periods of high pain became less destructive to their phenomenological self. Living with chronic pain meant that they had to continue to act in a way that is 'the new normal,' partly to avoid becoming an object of horror, disgust, and abjection due to their lack of control, but primarily to balance being in pain with everyday *functioning* – to put it simply, they still had to make dinner eventually. They had to find a way to experience the sensations of life and our sensations of self even as pain reduced their experience of the world, to integrate pain into their lives so that they are able to continue.

Despite this need to remake the self with pain, balancing pain in functioning is not wholly sustainable; pain must be given into. BDSM provides a space for giving in to pain;

> *That prickly pain of a slapped face. The deep ache of the next day, pulled muscles and all. That bruise that lingers for what seems like weeks. That can keep me*

going through the difficulties of the chronic pain. Chronic pain limits me, however much I try to believe otherwise, whereas kink pain frees me. Centers me in the moment, or the experience, or the continuing enduring effects thereof. That's why it matters.

(Julie, diary entry)

Julie's loss of control over her chronic pain came about because of a change in her disability. As a result of the loss of bodily capacity and capability from what she had grown used to, she had to stop the majority – and eventually all – of her BDSM play, which has meant that she has lost both an important source of pleasure, but also a large part of her phenomenological self;

Chronic pain was just a challenge to overcome. Since kink? This has allowed me to find a place to move away from the all encompassing pain/disability and just be me. Sure there are times when the chronic pain/disability have to play a part in the kink, I have major limitations, but to work beyond them is liberating. I've explored myself through the kink. Over the last few months I've lost a lot of confidence in my body as it has failed. My image of myself now includes my disability as a major component. I can't be the big and fun me any more, it's got lost in the pain for the time being. Having to hold onto to the hope I'll get "me" back.

(Julie, interview two)

This change to the lifeworld has led to Julie living in a period of mourning; she mourns the very real loss of her bodily capacity, but also the loss of her pain control method, and the loss of her lived experience, particularly as her preferred BDSM play space was a club – and therefore she has lost emotional and erotic relationships now the space is no longer accessible to her. As Julie points out, she no longer feels like herself; the change in her pain and fatigue levels has affected her phenomenological self – but she has not been wholly destroyed; she is instead going through a period of re-adjusting to her new self.

Charlie's experience of a change in pain and fatigue contrasted with Julie's, not because they are not experiencing a change in their phenomenological self, but because they are a little further on in their journey; the change is not so immediate, and there was less of a sense of mourning in how Charlie discussed the change in their lifeworld, even as they acknowledged the difficulty in adjusting;

Like I would have used it more in the past, it's been harder since the [diagnosis] and the more pain and just, my body's feeling less robust.

(Charlie, interview 1)

This difference may not be due just to time, however – it may be because Charlie's change in chronic pain is due to a *new* disability alongside the worsening of their original; it may be because Julie used BDSM as a primary method of pain control, while Charlie used it more for pleasure and re-establishing bodily ownership.

Charlie felt that there was a tension between their bodily response to pain in BDSM, and their cognitive function, explaining;

> *I noticed that I used to deal with my pain a lot through my mind, and I suppose now because the fatigue affects my cognitive function a bit, I don't have those mental resources to deal with the pain either.*
>
> (Charlie, interview 2)

Charlie's feeling that they lack the cognitive function to deal with their chronic pain – particularly the energy to focus their thoughts on anything other than pain, and thus resist the breakdown of self – is a feeling of a loss of control over their chronic pain, and a loss of control over the self.

It is this notion of control, control of the body and control of pain that has been particularly notable in my interviews, with participants seeking to find ways to not just regain a sense of control, but to regain their sense of self through exercising control over how they live with their pain. The world is at once shattered and held together through control, and finding a way to regain that sense of control is important to the re-establishment of the phenomenological self when living with chronic pain. BDSM, for most of the participants, was a key part of regaining that sense of control – but it also served other purposes. For Charlie, piercing and body modification are a part of their kink play,[8] and they practiced piercing and body modification as a part of reclaiming control over their body, particularly after their disabling accident;

> *And I know that [piercing and body modification] was about, sort of voluntary seeking pain, it was shortly after having been injured and having been living with disability and chronic pain, so it was all about my body in voluntary, more positive kind of ways, um, I supposed maiming it in voluntary ways and experiencing the pain in sort of, a controlled situation.*
>
> (Charlie, interview 1)

These practices are painful – involving a deliberate breaking of skin, although they are not intended to cause long-term *harm* – and for Charlie, the practices were a pleasurable and positive re-establishment of selfhood, and of their "ownership" of their body. This ownership is also expressed by participants in terms of self-awareness, of knowing their bodily capacities and limits, and how pain affects those capacities;

> *sometimes it's okay to just be with it, but also learning to listen to your body so that you can... so that you can manage it more.... But also understanding what your body's saying as well, because there is that balance, that I thought, if I just... If I just went into my fatigue, I wouldn't get off the sofa ever, or something. You know? But you have to then figure out what are the times when you can try and work with... you know, continue through it, or when you do just have to sit with it.... Because you could just sit with it all the time and do nothing, but there's also the*

> *danger of going the other way and trying to push through it when you're not going to be able to get through it. It's just going to make it worse. So it's about staying active in a way that is sustainable, or is safe, that is not going to have the same... But you can't always predict it.*
>
> (Charlie, interview 2)

This awareness is a part of control, in that it is necessary to know when control is possible – and when pushing oneself to the limit of one's capacity is possible, or necessary. Charlie, like other participants, used their self-awareness to decide when and how to play, but as Julie explained, self-awareness is in itself painful, because it requires being aware of pain; there is a tension for all participants between enough self-awareness to engage with the world and the self, and experiencing pain so much that it becomes overwhelming. Thus, control of awareness becomes necessary, and for Julie, this is a conscious process;

> *I can't now remember what it's like not to have [chronic pain] there, um ... and as such I cope by kind of, by not being in tune with my body at all, um, and basically by living in my head... which is fine until I break a leg or something and I don't notice [laughs]... –so I don't, I kind of stop taking any signals from my body, because it's just, yeah, if all I'm getting back is 'that hurts, everything hurts' type stuff, I just kind of have to go through it all..., I'm often completely unaware of when my body is massively complaining because – because I'm not listening to it.*
>
> (Julie, interview 1)

This awareness – this refusal to let the phenomenological self shatter under pain – is not necessarily conscious, or deliberate; it is a part of living with chronic pain.

Self-Control and Containment

Control is not always possible – or wanted, and thus we turn here to the deliberate *loss* of control, the controlled uncontrolled spaces of kink, and the uncontrolled spaces of loss.

Charlie identified the notion of control as an important part of living with chronic pain – but particularly the discourse of *self*-control, that to perform proper bodily humanness, a person must perform proper control;

CHARLIE: *"well, it's about control again, isn't it? This idea of we're supposed to be in control.... Something you can't control and it just sort of spills out."*
INTERVIEWER: *"yeah. So a space for it to spill out is sometimes..."*
CHARLIE: *"useful... and welcome and wanted. Sought out" (Charlie, interview 2).*

Charlie went on to explain that pain is sometimes reacted to as though it were a bodily fluid – one that should be properly contained within the body, and certainly not allowed to leak out in the view of others;

> *[pain] doesn't necessarily impact on people in the sense that you're not going to piss on somebody's seat with your pain, but... so it's slightly different, but... so in some ways, there's even less scope for it to spill out, because people don't see it when it does.*
>
> (Charlie, interview 2)

This need for bodily containment is echoed in discourses of 'leaky' bodies, particularly bodies which menstruate, the incontinence of very young or very old bodies, and the incontinence of disabled bodies (Liddiard and Slater, 2017). As discussed in the previous chapter, failure to contain leaks – failure to keep uncontrollable leaks private – is incompatible with proper bodymindedness, and a failure of proper self-control. Expressing pain works as a leak because it is horrifying, abject, and could be particularly significant for Charlie, as a trans person, because leaking is feminizing (and thus also horrifying to the observer, as a signifier of leaking femininity). Expressions of pain are reacted to in the same way as leaks of physical fluids, as though observing/acknowledging the expression of pain will make that pain contagious – will cause the observer to feel that pain.

Kink is both a space to forgo control, and to express pain, but also served as a space in which to relieve the social pressure to contain responses to pain. This echoes discourses of submission as relief from high-stress, high-responsibility employment (Newmahr, 2011; Weiss, 2011) – the proverbial submissive man as successful businessman by day, kinky submissive by night – but for the participants, this discourse is used to create space for submission and receiving pain as relief from chronic pain and self-control. Julie exemplified this, explaining

> *I'm known for being efficient, i think i control as much of life as i can (and others if given half the chance, in my professional life that is). Part of my kink is submission, giving that control to someone else in some ways, and letting them control my pain levels. That giving over of control is really important to me.*
>
> (Julie, interview 2)

Julie used kink to create a space where she felt it was safe to engage with her body – where she could allow herself to fully experience her chronic pain, which she otherwise pushed to the back of her mind. In addition, she felt that kink was a positive experience of pain, compared to chronic pain. She explained that when she experiences her highest pain, she finds it overwhelming;

> *i long for release, to finally feel myself pass out from the pain is often such a relief. I'd rather not know how much I'm hurting, even when bedbound from pain, because then it is more 'real'/overwhelming/large component of my life.*
>
> (Julie, interview 2)

The sensation of kink pain played an important part in control and engaging with the body, for several participants. As Natalie explained, kink is a reminder of the capacities of her body, rather than the limitations she is often faced with due to fatigue, which are often frustratingly unpredictable due to the reliably unreliability of her chronic illness. In 'taking' a spanking, or engaging in rough play, and therefore enduring the acute pain that results, Natalie is able to re-establish her body as capable;

> *It also makes my body feel stronger; i tense up, and absorb the impact [of being spanked] and that sort of strength, maybe endurance, makes me feel good.*
>
> (Natalie interview two)

This does not mean that kink sex is the only method of re-establishing a sense of bodily capacity available to chronically ill or disabled people; it is one that Natalie enjoys, while others may prefer more 'vanilla' sex, a sport, or a more sedentary hobby. The important factor is one of a capacity for *pleasure*, rather than endurance or pain.

The sensation of pain itself, as already discussed, is tightly controlled within kink play, as only particular instruments or methods of pain creation are used once the scene has been agreed upon, and therefore, as Michelle explained, the pain from play can feel very different to the already present chronic pain;

> *it's different to the pain that's already in my body, and i think that's what makes it bearable, in a way.*
>
> (Michelle interview 1)

This difference in sensation is still understood as 'pain' with a strict medical interpretation – a triggering of receptors and a firing of neurons – but a broader interpretation of these sensations gives a very different understanding, one that is dependent on context and intent as well as social constructions of pain itself. The difference in sensation is important to Julie, who explains that:

> *The focusing pain calms me, the sensations aren't as deep and pervasive as in chronic pain, the pain is specific. I can appreciate it changing sensations, the pain peaking and troughing. I react in many ways to kink pain, it invigorates me, it turns me on, it allows me to breathe deep full happy breaths. My body doesn't cope very well to non-kink, non-chronic pain, it tends to exaggerate the sensations, making a papercut seem highly painful. It goes into shut down mode quite quickly in these situations.*
>
> (Julie, interview 2)

The context of pain is particularly important to Julie; that she has consented to pain does not make it less *painful*, because, as she explains, living with chronic pain has made her more sensitive to pain – an experience described in medicine as 'priming,' whereby the receptors and neurons involved in sensing pain are already close to being triggered due to chronic pain, and thus relatively minor events are felt more strongly (Denk et al., 2014). However, a strictly medical understanding would make Julie *less* inclined to engage in kink; the assumed aversive nature of pain experience would conclude that she would find kink too painful to engage in, especially as she is 'primed' to experience higher levels of pain. That Julie describes the sensation as pain means that it is pain – but a form of painful sensation which is not aversive, and is, for Julie, positive – invigorating, arousing, calming – and helps her to engage with her body.

In re-engaging with pain as sensation, participants used kink to speak back to pain, as well as welcoming sensation; they are using the capacities of their bodies to bring them pleasure, and to have a positive experience of pain. As Catherine explains;

> *there's that thing where chronic pain … it becomes extremely negative and extremely like there's a feeling of just tiredness associated with it and kind of often getting to the end of your tether with it and… a very negative relationship and possibly that having a negative effect on… on being in your body, like i was saying…. But the emotions i associate with pain in kink are sort of stimulation especially. Much less of a sense of inconvenience because if anything seems wrong then i can ask for it to be stopped…. And, like, everything else can be shut out and i can be very, very present. Which is… is… yeah, presumably other people who are not kinky find that in other places, other things. And yeah, it's much more of a sort of malleable thing that i can make work for me and that is sort of very positive.*
>
> (Catherine, interview 1)

The idea of making her pain work for her – controlling pain and how it is experienced, rather than pain dominating her actions – is an important part of Catherine's chosen way of controlling pain, alongside more normative pain control methods. For Natalie, inducing pain through kink worked for her in another way;

> *i have very low blood pressure and can faint when i orgasm (when things are bad, i can faint when i sneeze!). This is a little dangerous, but it is also psychologically unpleasant and trigger the scant remains of my PTSD. Erotic pain is something which can help keep me conscious.*
>
> (Natalie, interview 1)

Several participants brought up that they were using kink pain in multiple ways, having consciously thought through their reasons for engaging with kink, and with pain play in particular – this is not unusual, as self-awareness is largely deemed (by kink communities) important for engaging in kink; for my participants, it was also an important part of living with chronic pain. For some of the participants, pain play could serve, very literally, as pain relief – as Charlie explained;

> *In any sort of kink or sex kind of play … sometimes [they]'ve been able to, uh, extend the period between using analgesia because of the impact of the endorphins, and just, whatever.*
>
> (Charlie, interview one)

Charlie identified flogging and needle play in particular as having an effect on pain sensation. They explained that this meant having pain caused in a particular area (away from the original injury site) as a part of play, which in turn helped to dull the sharper sensation they feel due to nerve damage around the injury site. This could also be combined with what they called "*desensitization work*," (Charlie, interview two), a gentler, therapeutic touch on the areas of nerve damage;

> *The desensitization work was secondary to the pain play, and relied on the biochemical and whole-body feeling changes of the preceding pain play to be explored.*
> (Charlie, interview three)

For Charlie, desensitization work was a methodological, carefully thought out, and purposeful use of kink pain to help them live with their chronic pain. This use of pain in pain management is not unheard of, although percussion treatment for painful amputation stumps is practiced much less than it was in the mid-20th century (Bourke, 2014). Natalie also reported that orgasm from sex (whether including kink or not) gave her a measure of temporary pain relief, and sex with kink resulted in stronger orgasms, and thus more effective relief – although it was also more tiring for her, meaning it was more costly in terms of fatigue afterwards. Rita also experienced a measure of pain relief from kink play;

> *[the pain] aches less, primarily. I think often because I've been maybe in the sort of very relaxed headspace, possibly my muscles are more relaxed or… but sometimes it feels like the one pain has driven out the other, and then once the… once the kink pain has started to fade, there's still less of the existing pain.*
> (Rita, interview 1)

For other participants, kink pain could overlay – not quite replace – chronic pain; in its urgency and acute sensation, it pulled attention away from chronic pain. Acute pain in a controlled situation allowed for a control of pain, again welcoming in sensation, reshaping the context. Edward explained that kink play more generally – not just pain from play – could act as a distraction, taking his mind off of his pain temporarily, as he was focused on performing tasks for his mistress. This drawing of focus away from chronic pain was also experienced by Charlie, who explained when asked why they liked kink;

> *It becomes very – so whilst i can enjoy the sensation, but sometimes i can also hate the sensation, but – enjoying hating it sometimes as well. But also, it – it does become that focus, it takes away from – i suppose other pain in some ways.*
> (Charlie, interview 2)

This, combined with the feeling of having successfully endured the scene, was what Charlie identified as their main reason for engaging in kink. The combination of forcing attention away from pain, but within a space where pain can also be reacted to and made public may seem contradictory, but the two processes work side-by-side by creating pain that must be reacted to, pulling the focus away from *containment* and onto expression – and thus into relief. This is particularly important for Catherine, who struggles to push her focus away from her pain;

> *i would say that I'm not very good at the consciously pushing-away part. If it's happening semi-automatically, i think I'm really good at it. As soon as it's hard to deal with, i end up going for painkillers (or alcohol if it's in the evening, or just going to sleep, or what have you).*
>
> (Catherine, interview 2)

While kink play can be read as a space to reclaim normal humanity through enacting and controlling pain, kink is outside of normative sexuality, and therefore normal humanity cannot be reclaimed by engaging in kink. However, the participants felt themselves to be already outside of the normal human because of their disabilities and chronic pain; they cannot reclaim normal humanity without becoming non-disabled; the ideal of able-bodymindedness and normative sexuality is forever beyond their reach. Their decision – and desire – to engage in kink play is instead a performance of abnormality, a performance of queer/crip sexuality. Several of the participants felt that being disabled made it easier for them to engage in non-normative sexual practices – including kink, but also having polyamorous relationships – because they are already cast as abnormal, and they have no desire to become normal, to be rehabilitated. Just as the non-disabled cannot perceive of themselves as disabled[9] (Hughes, 2012; Kumari Campbell, 2009a; Wendell, 1996), disabled people cannot perceive of themselves as non-disabled, except in the past; I would not be *myself* if I were not disabled, as my bodily experience of chronic pain and disability has shaped who I am, shaped my phenomenological self. Kink exposes being normal as not just impossible, but also as *unwanted* – and for participants, embracing abnormality is not just possible, but necessary. Thus, in deciding not to strive for normality – to not fall in with the societal push for rehabilitation – the participants are re-establishing their phenomenological self, controlling their pain – or not controlling it – as they choose, rather than just when, and how, control is required, performing normality when it is useful, when being read as normal gives them an advantage (although as discussions of pity and others' readings of their bodies showed, participants sometimes performed normality at unexpected times) – and then performing abnormality when they felt comfortable or safe to do so, or when being abnormal is advantageous.

Making Pain

Through engaging in kink, the participants are engaging in a process of *making pain to witness*, of making pain visible through participating in acts that are deliberately painful – in contrast to their chronic pain, which has no witness. Making pain is an act of meaningful communication (Price, 2015), but in making pain to be witnessed, to be seen and heard by another, they are drawing the witnesses into their pain, as "the act of witnessing somebody else's pain … is a performative act that affects all involved bodies, both in and out of pain" (Kolářová, 2010: 47). Making pain to witness is both a part of controlling the expression of, and reaction to, pain, but also a part of integrating pain into the self.

Communicating about pain is a part of making pain to witness – for those participants who found their chronic pain impacted their capacities for play (such as how long they could play for, or what form that play could take), communicating pain plays a dual role; they are communicating their play pain, and also their chronic pain. This is not to say communication is always straightforward, as Natalie explained;

> *Because we both have chronic pain, we're able to communicate about pain pretty well, and have gradually become more explicit, even though our descriptions are often quite gruesome. With [husband]'s pain, i often try and pin him down to a number between one in ten, but i really struggle to do that with myself.*
>
> (Natalie, interview 1)

The number system Natalie refers to is an informal variation of the Wong-Baker scale (Wong et al., 2001), and while quantifying pain may make it a little easier for her to understand, as her own and her husband's responses show, it is often difficult for the person in pain to do in a way they are satisfied with. Making pain to talk about – pain that is easier to express, and thus easier to experience – aids in this communication, as it is a different experience of pain, an expansion of the vocabulary of pain and a point of comparison, and also a shared experience between the person in pain and the person causing that pain.

Notes

1 Inevitably, as the discourse of self-control has grown out of the asylum discourse.
2 Examining this discourse – which equates becoming ill with personal failure – is perhaps at the root of resistance to including chronic illness in disability – disability activists have long sought to distance themselves from both medical discourses and discourses of blame, and illness only reintroduces these.
3 Organic over non-organic, fresh over frozen, 'homecooked' over 'pre-prepared,' and so on and so forth.
4 While using the political language of Black feminist activism, which names self-care as a political act (Ahmed, 2014; Lorde, 1988).
5 See Chapter 4.
6 Your own mileage here may vary.
7 It should be noted that some drugs usually prescribed as antidepressants can also act as muscle relaxers, which can reduce pain levels, for some people – but I refer here to depression tied to living with chronic pain.
8 Body modification and piercing are not necessarily considered a part of BDSM, although they can be; in Charlie's life the two activities are connected.
9 See previous chapter.

References

Adelson N (2010) The Fit of Heath: Embodied Health Ideals and Its Implications. In: Lange I and Norridge Z (eds) *Illness, Bodies and Contexts: Interdisciplinary Perspectives*. Oxford: Inter-disciplinary Press, pp. 49–56.

Ahmed S (2014) Selfcare as Warfare. Available at: http://feministkilljoys.com/2014/08/25/selfcare-as-warfare/ (accessed 29 May 2015).

Bourke J (2014) *The Story of Pain: From Prayer to Painkillers*. Oxford: Oxford University Press.

Braidotti R (2011) *Nomadic Subjects: Embodiment and Sexual Difference in Contemporary Feminist Theory*. 2nd ed. New York: Columbia University Press.

Cooper C (2010) Fat Studies: Mapping the Field: Fat Studies. *Sociology Compass* 4(12): 1020–1034. DOI: 10.1111/j.1751–9020.2010.00336.x.

de Wolfe P (2002) Private Tragedy in Social Context? Reflections on Disability, Illness and Suffering. *Disability & Society* 17(3): 255–267.

Denk F, McMahon SB and Tracey I (2014) Pain Vulnerability: A Neurobiological Perspective. *Nature Neuroscience* 17(2): 192–200. DOI: 10.1038/nn.3628.

Garland-Thomson R (2009) *Staring: How We Look*. Oxford: New York: Oxford University Press.

Goffman E (2006) Selections from Stigma. In: Davies LJ (ed) *The Disability Studies Reader*. 2nd ed. Abingdon: Routledge, pp. 131–140.

Gordon A (2020) *What We Don't Talk about When We Talk about Fat*. Boston, MA: Beacon Press.

Grosz EA (1994) *Volatile Bodies: Towards a Corporeal Feminism*. Bloomington: Indiana University Press.

Hughes B (2012) Civilising Modernity and the Ontological Invalidation of Disabled People. In: Goodley D, Hughes B and Davis L (eds) *Disability and Social Theory: New Developments and Directions*. Abingdon: Palgrave Macmillan, pp. 17–32.

Kafer A (2013) *Feminist, Queer, Crip*. Bloomington and Indianapolis: Indiana University Press.

Kolářová K (2010) Performing the Pain: Opening the (Crip) Body for (Queer) Pleasures. *Review of Disability Studies* 6(3): 44–52.

Kristeva J (1997) Powers of Horror (abridged). In: Oliver K (ed) *The Portable Kristeva*. 2nd ed. New York: Columbia University Press, pp. 229–263.

Kumari Campbell F (2009a) *Contours of Ableism: The Production of Disability and Abledness*. Basingstoke: Palgrave Macmillan.

Kumari Campbell F (2009b) Having a Career in Disability Studies Without Even Becoming Disabled! The Strains of the Disabled Teaching Body. *International Journal of Inclusive Education* 13(7): 713–725. DOI: 10.1080/13603110903046002.

Langdridge D (2007) Speaking the Unspeakable: S/M & the Eroticisation of Pain. In: Barker M and Langdridge D (eds) *Safe, Sane & Consensual: Contemporary Perspectives of Sadomasochism*. Basingstoke: Palgrave Macmillan, pp. 85–97.

Liddiard K and Slater J (2017) 'Like, Pissing Yourself Is Not the Most Attractive Quality, Let's be Honest': Learning to Contain Through Youth, Adulthood, Disability and Sexuality. *Sexualities* 21(3): 319–333. DOI: 10.1177/1363460716688674.

Lorde A (1988) *A Burst of Light, Essays*. London: Sheba Feminist Publishers.

McRuer R (2006) *Crip Theory: Cultural Signs of Queerness and Disability*. New York: NYU Press.

Miller WI (1997) *The Anatomy of Disgust*. Cambridge, MA: Harvard University Press.

Newmahr S (2011) *Playing on the Edge: Sadomasochism, Risk, and Intimacy*. Bloomington: Indiana University Press.

Nielsen A and Fernandez J (2010) Journeys with Chronic Pain: Acquiring Stigma Along the Way. In: Fernandez J (ed) *Making Sense of Pain: Critical and Interdisciplinary Perspectives*. Oxford: Inter-Disciplinary Press, pp. 45–54.

Price M (2015) The Bodymind Problem and the Possibilities of Pain. *Hypatia* 30(1): 268–284. DOI: 10.1111/hypa.12127.

Scarry E (1985) *The Body in Pain: The Making and Unmaking of the World*. New York: Oxford University Press.

Shildrick M (2009) *Dangerous Discourses of Disability, Subjectivity and Sexuality*. Basingstoke: Palgrave Macmillan.

Sumpter S (2012) The Paralympics Tell Us Nothing about Most Sick or Disabled People. Available at: http://www.latentexistence.me.uk/the-paralympics-tell-us-nothing-about-most-sick-or-disabled-people/ (accessed 12 September 2012).

Thomas SP and Johnson M (2000) A Phenomenologic Study of Chronic Pain. *Western Journal of Nursing Research* 22(6): 683–705.

Tremain S (ed) (2005) *Foucault and the Government of Disability*. Ann Arbor: University of Michigan Press.

Tyler I (2013) *Revolting Subjects: Social Abjection and Resistance in Neoliberal Britain*. London: Zed Books.

Waldschmidt A (2005) Who Is Normal? Who Is Deviant? 'Normality' and 'Risk' in Genetic Diagnostics and Counselling. In: Tremain S (ed.) *Foucault and the Government of Disability*. Ann Arbor: University of Michigan Press, pp. 191–207.

Weiss M (2011) *Techniques of Pleasure: BDSM and the Circuits of Sexuality*. Durham, NC and London: Duke University Press.

Wendell S (1996) *The Rejected Body: Feminist Philosophical Reflections on Disability*. New York: Routledge.

Williams SJ and Bendelow G (1998) *The Lived Body: Sociological Themes, Embodied Issues*. Abingdon: Routledge.

Wong DL, Hockenberry-Eaton M, Wilson D, et al. (2001) Wong-Baker FACES Pain Scale. In: *Wong's Essentials of Pediatric Nursing*. 6th edn. St Louise, MO: Mosby, p. 1301.

Young S (2012) We're Not Here for Your Inspiration. Available at: http://www.abc.net.au/news/2012-07-03/young-inspiration-porn/4107006 (accessed 12 September 2012).

Conclusion

Through this book, I have made a few big claims. Firstly: ableism and compulsory ableness structure and constrain how we understand pain within and outside of medicine; there is a distinction between pain and long-term chronic pain (as a disability) which is missing. In effect, ableist discourse expects all pain to be the same – in particular, that pain is negative, unwanted, and ontologically impossible in the long-term. A critical crip theory approach illuminates the discourses at work here; the cripistemologies of people living with chronic pain which emerged in my participants' narratives demonstrated particular crip knowledge/understanding of what it is to live with chronic pain. In particular, we see that living with chronic pain – and in particular how that is shaped through the demands of normative expectations of everyday life – produces particular ways of living in and living through crip time.

Exploring chronic pain alongside BDSM might seem like an odd choice, at first. However, non-normative and queer sexualities (in which I include kink/BDSM) and disabled people's sexualities and sexual practices have a great deal of overlap and parallels – and who better to ask about pain than people who have lived with pain for years, but still deliberately choose to experience *more pain*. In exploring how they experience both kink and chronic pain, and what kink brings to their lives, we see a range of experiences and engagements with kink and pain. Normative sociocultural expectations of what pain is, and particularly the stigma having pain while living in a pain-averse (or analgesic) culture, means that participants felt pushed to ignore their pain; kink was used by them as a way to engage with bodily sensation, including pain.

In addition, pain-averse sociocultural expectations of the normal bodymind mean that in order to be recognized as normal – to not be abject – the bodymind must be controlled. In this regard pain functions as a bodily fluid; it must be contained and not expressed within view of others (either in public or private). This is one of the key drivers of participants feeling pushed to ignore or minimize their pain. Kink, for some participants, made a space in which they gained a sense of control over their pain. For others, kink was used as a way of making space/time to be uncontrolled – to express their pain and have their expression recognized by others.

DOI: 10.4324/9781003006237-7

Index

Note: Page numbers followed by "n" denote endnotes.

For Product Safety Concerns and Information please contact our
EU representative GPSR@taylorandfrancis.com Taylor & Francis
Verlag GmbH, Kaufingerstraße 24, 80331 München, Germany